Alpha Pamela Sanchéz Valle
Marcela Autran Martínez
Gabriel Eduardo Acevedo Jiménez

The immune response of the cat to FeLV infection

Alpha Pamela Sanchéz Valle
Marcela Autran Martínez
Gabriel Eduardo Acevedo Jiménez

The immune response of the cat to FeLV infection

Immune response to different types of feline viral leukemia virus infection

ScienciaScripts

Imprint

Cover image: www.ingimage.com

This book is a translation from the original published under ISBN 978-613-9-41116-0.

Publisher:
Sciencia Scripts
is a trademark of
Dodo Books Indian Ocean Ltd. and OmniScriptum S.R.L publishing group

120 High Road, East Finchley, London, N2 9ED, United Kingdom
Str. Armeneasca 28/1, office 1, Chisinau MD-2012, Republic of Moldova, Europe
Printed at: see last page
ISBN: 978-620-8-11351-3

The cat's immune response to feline viral leukaemia virus infection

Alpha Pamela Sanchez Valle

Dr. Marcela Autran Martínez

Dr. Gabriel Eduardo Acevedo Jiménez

INDEX

1. SUMMARY 4
2. INTRODUCTION 6
3. OBJECTIVES 9
3.1. GENERAL OBJECTIVE 9
3.2. PARTICULAR OBJECTIVE 9
4. JUSTIFICATION 10
5. MATERIALS AND METHODS 11
6. LITERATURE REVIEW 12
6.1. EVOLUTION OF THE VIRUS 12
6.2. DISCOVERY 12
6.3. GENETIC STRUCTURE 12
6.4. FeLV GENETIC DIVERSITY 15
6.4.1. ENDOGENIC FORM OF FeLV 15
6.4.2. EXOGENOUS FORM OF FeLV 16
6.4.2.1. SUB-GROUP A 18
6.4.2.2. SUB-GROUP B 18
6.4.2.3. SUB-GROUP C 18
6.4.2.4. SUB-GROUP T 19
6.4.2.5. NEW SUB-GROUPS 19
6.5. TRANSMISSION 19
6.6. COURSE OF INFECTION 21
6.7. IMMUNE RESPONSE TO FeLV VIRUS 24
6.7.1. INNATE IMMUNITY 26
6.7.1.1. INTEGUMENTARY SYSTEM 26
6.7.1.5. PHYSICAL AND CHEMICAL FACTORS 32
6.7.1.6. MOLECULAR FACTORS 39
6.7.1.6.1.4. INTERFERON 42
6.7.1.6.1.5. TOLL-LIKE RECEPTORS (TLR) 43
6.7.1.6.1.6. MAJOR HISTOCOMPATIBILITY COMPLEX (MHC) 44
6.7.1.7. CELLULAR FACTORS 44
6.7.1.7.1.4. CYTOTOXIC CELLS 46
6.7.2. ORGANS AND CELLS OF THE IMMUNE RESPONSE 47
6.7.2.1. PRIMARY: THYMUS, BONE MARROW 48

6.7.2.1.1. TIMO 48
6.7.2.1.2. BONE MARROW 48
6.7.2.2. LYMPHOID ORGANS 49
6.7.2.2.1. LYMPHONODS 49
6.7.2.2.2. CHEST 49
6.7.3. CELL-MEDIATED IMMUNITY 50
6.7.3.1. HUMORAL IMMUNITY 50
6.7.4. DIAGNOSTIC TESTS 52
6.7.5. FELV-ASSOCIATED VIRAL ONCOGENESIS 55
6.7.6. VACCINES AND VACCINATION 57
6.7.6.1. FACTORS TO CONSIDER IN ESTABLISHING A VACCINATION SCHEDULE 57
6.7.6.2. VACCINES AVAILABLE IN MEXICO 58
6.7.6.3. SUGGESTIONS FOR A VACCINATION PROTOCOL 60
7. CONCLUSION 62
8. REFERENCES 63

1. SUMMARY

In this study, a literature review of the immune response to feline viral leukaemia virus (FeLV) infection was carried out and information was collected on various aspects of the humoral and cellular immune response as a result of the cat's interaction with the FeLV virus. The immune response must be effective and specific from the moment the cat comes into contact with the virus. Cellular and humoral immunity are responsible for controlling the infection and each has its own way of acting against the virus, as antibodies are known to stop the spread of the virus and establish resistance to infection, Cellular immunity is responsible for the elimination of already infected cells and protects against the development of latent infection, so the quality and magnitude of both will determine the course of infection, however, retroviruses can alter these mechanisms, as they infect mainly lymphocytes and cells from the bone marrow, altering their function; However, the outcome of the interaction with the virus is not based solely on the immune response, as virus-specific factors such as subtype and viral concentration can influence the outcome; If the immune response is effective and there is low exposure to FeLV, replication of the virus can be stopped and there is no viraemia, or the virus can be isolated and replicate in a single tissue, resulting in an abortive or focal infection, the late but effective immune response, where the virus does not infect bone marrow and viraemia is terminated, will result in a regressive infection, where the virus is not eliminated but remains latent and at risk of reactivation in the event of an immunosuppressive event; if the immune system has a poor response or is absent, the host develops a progressive infection with persistent viraemia and development of FeLV-associated diseases which can be fatal. There is no specific treatment to treat patients with FeLV, however, rFeINF-ω is used in infected cats and is theorised to modulate the innate response and affect the FeLV replication cycle. The virus affects a variety of apparatus and systems in the cat's body and will present with different diseases, the most common of which is the development of tumours, which have been described in various organs of infected cats. The extent to which FeLV may be involved in the development of tumours in FeLV-negative patients is not yet known, as immunohistochemical tests are not commonly performed in these patients. It is common in clinical practice that POC tests are performed on healthy and sick cats, however, a positive or negative result is not the end of the diagnosis, as it must be taken into account that there may be an error in the test, in addition the risk factors of each individual must be considered, for this reason it is recommended to repeat the test or perform PCR to determine if the cat is infected and if so, to know what is the course of infection. Knowing the retroviral status and risk factors of the cat will help us to establish an individualised immunological status and vaccination schedule in order to provide protection to the cat.

2. INTRODUCTION

The immune system is one of the most complex and diverse components of a living being and its primary purpose is to provide protection against the variety of infectious agents responsible for morbidity and mortality; it is capable of responding, with varying degrees of effectiveness, to bacterial, viral, fungal, protozoan and helminthic pathogens. The immune system is composed of specialised effector cells that sense and respond to foreign cells, antigens, and other molecular patterns not found in tissues (Barret et al., 2016)The immune system is involved in inflammatory and tissue repair processes and can initiate responses to abnormal cells that arise during neoplastic transformation or that may be inappropriately transplanted into the body. Such a potent biological system requires careful management and a comprehensive set of regulatory mechanisms to ensure that immune responses are inactivated when not needed, so that they do not cause unintended damage to normal body tissue. (Day & Schultz, 2014). Among domestic animals, the immune system of the dog and cat has only been examined in detail in relatively recent times; the dog as a model for transplant surgery, and the cat as a model for the study of virus-induced neoplasia (feline leukaemia virus [FeLV]) or immunodeficiency (feline immunodeficiency virus [FIV]), have led to the application of cellular and molecular techniques to characterise basic facets of the immune system (Day, 2012).

Infections caused by feline retroviruses cause profound imbalances in the immune system, as they are viruses that mainly infect lymphocytes and cells of different lineages from the bone marrow, altering their functionality. (Porras M, 2007).

FeLV is a retrovirus of the genus *Gammaretrovirus* that affects all domestic cats worldwide. Its viral structure consists of an envelope, core and nucleocapsid. All retrovirus genomes contain three genes called *gag*, *pol* and *env* (gp70 and p15e), which encode proteins that are very important for the virus. (Palmero & Carballés Pérez, 2010)..

In domestic cats (*Felis catus*) FeLV has been classified based on evidence of interference, viral neutralisation and ability to replicate in non-cat tissues, into three main subgroups: A, B, C and a fourth group-T; recently associated with T lymphocytes and related to immunodeficiency processes due to its tropism towards lymphocyte receptors; of all the subgroups mentioned, FeLV subgroup A (FeLV-A) is the only one contagious from cat to cat in the wild. (Calle R et al., 2013; Collado A, 2017) that has been described so far.

The pathogenesis of FeLV is very complex and unlike feline immunodeficiency (FIV), the evolution of FeLV is strongly influenced by the cat's immune response capacity, and FeLV can even be eliminated in early stages of infection. (Porras M, 2007).

The immune response to FeLV develops after viral exposure, however, the host maintains a delicate balance between virus and cell, leading to host resistance to persistent infection. Most cats exposed to FeLV develop a temporary infection, with or without transient viraemia, and either recover completely or establish latent infection. Both humoral and cell-mediated immune responses are important for controlling infection (Mizayawa, 2002).

Normally, the humoral response develops in the first weeks (4th-8th) post infection, in this response the anti-gp70 antibody is subgroup specific and results in viral neutralisation and immunity to reinfection by preventing virus binding to the cellular receptor. (Calle R et al., 2013; Porras M, 2007).. On the other hand, the p15 protein has been shown to interfere with the host's cellular immune response and thus facilitate viral persistence. Recently it has been described that its immunosuppressive function is of great importance *in vivo*, even inhibiting the proper development of post-vaccination humoral immunity (Adams et al., 1979; Calle R et al., 2013). . A non-viral protein detected in FeLV infection is the FOCMA antigen (*Feline Oncornavirus Cell Membrane Antigen*); in some cats this protein is expressed on the surface of infected and malignant B or T lymphocytes (lymphosarcoma); the immune system is able to recognise this protein, form protective antibodies and destroy the cells that express it, thus reducing the likelihood of developing lymphocyte tumours, but not other disease-related conditions (Collado A, 2017). (Collado A, 2017).

The cellular immune response is also necessary for the control of viral replication and elimination, and cytotoxic CD8+ T lymphocytes have been shown to appear one to two weeks after infection and prior to the appearance of neutralising antibodies (Mizayawa, 2002; Porras M., 2007). (Mizayawa, 2002; Porras M, 2007)..

antibodies (Mizayawa, 2002; Porras M., 2007). (Mizayawa, 2002; Porras M, 2007)..

3. OBJECTIVES

3.1. GENERAL OBJECTIVE

To compile a compendium of relevant scientific information to explain and describe all possible aspects involved in the immune response of cats to FeLV infection, allowing a broader view of the different factors involved in this disease.

3.2. PARTICULAR PURPOSE

Collect available information on the host/host-host interaction of cats that come into contact with FeLV, describe the possible outcomes of the cat's interaction with the virus, as well as methods to properly diagnose the course of infection; compile the most common conditions observed in infected patients and propose a FeLV vaccination schedule based on the risk factors for each cat, in order to allow other clinicians to consult this research and the literature sources cited, to gain a better understanding of the disease and perhaps continue the work done.

4. JUSTIFICATION

This literature review will provide us with a compendium of information about the interaction between the virus and the cat's immune system, understanding how the immune response is triggered, which cells and molecules are involved, and how these interactions influence the course of the disease, as this is essential for the development of prevention and diagnostic strategies for a viral disease that is highly contagious and is a major cause of illness and death in cats.

5. MATERIALS AND METHODS

A series of consecutive procedures were carried out in accordance with the scientific method applied to a documentary review, including the selection of the topic, planning of the work, collection of information and writing of the research paper, according to what is described in the index ; collecting scientific information from books, main sources and biomedical databases. The most relevant articles and documents related to the topic of this research were used.

6. LITERATURE REVIEW

6.1. EVOLUTION OF THE VIRUS

In 1975, Benveniste, Sherr and Todaro, conducted a study that showed that FeLV-related gene sequences are found only in the cellular DNA of four members of the genus *Felidae*, namely the pathogen-specific free domestic cat (*Felis catus*), the jungle cat (*F. chaus*), the sand cat (*F. margarita*) and the European wild cat (*F. sylvestris*). (Willet & Hoise, 2013)It is theorised that these genes were introduced following trans-species infection with a rodent *Gammaretrovirus*, as the cellular DNA of these contains related virogenic sequences (Benveniste et al., 1975).. Retroviral genes can be naturally transferred between related mammals, incorporated into their germ lines and inherited as cellular genes (Benveniste & Todaro, 1975). (Benveniste & Todaro, 1982)..

6.2. DISCOVERY

In 1964, William Jarrett and co-workers observed histopathological findings of murine leukaemia virus-like particles in the lymphosarcoma of a cat living in a cattery where the animals developed malignant lymphomas, thus discovering FeLV, and tumours were thought to be the main consequence of FeLV infection, but it is now known that this is one of many manifestations that FeLV can cause. (Crawford et al., 1964; News, 2019)..

6.3. GENETIC STRUCTURE

FeLV is an 8.3 kb single-stranded linear RNA molecule retrovirus that belongs to the *Retroviridae* family of the genus *Gammaretrovirus* (Guliukina et al., 2019; Neil, 2010).. All retrovirus genomes contain three essential genes called *gag*, *pol* and *env* that encode proteins important for the virus, flanked by long terminal repeats (LTRs) at each end and possess the information necessary for the initiation and termination of gene expression, the LTR of leukaemia viruses, plays a critical role in tissue tropism and pathogenic potential of the viruses (Abujamra et al., 2006).. The *gag* (group-specific antigen) gene carries the information necessary to encode the internal structural proteins of the virus, p15 (matrix protein, MA), p12 (unknown function), p27 (capsid protein, CA) and p10 nucleocapsid protein, NC); the *pol* (polymerase) gene encodes proteins with enzymatic activity required for viral replication, p14 (protease, PR), p80 (reverse transcriptase, RT) and p46 (integrase, IN) and the *env* (envelope) gene encodes the different components of the envelope, gp70 (surface unit, SU) and p15e (transmembrane proteins, TM) that affect normal lymphocyte function (**Figure 1**). (Mizayawa, 2002). The gp70 glycoprotein determines the three main FeLV subgroups: A, B and C and is involved in the induction of specific immunity, as it is the main target of the humoral immune response (Willet & Hoise, 2013). (Willet & Hoise, 2013).

The FeLV viral structure consists of an envelope, core and nucleocapsid. In the core is the single-stranded RNA, which upon introduction into host cells is transcribed into DNA, which is integrated into the host genome with the help of the enzyme reverse transcriptase, once a DNA copy of the RNA genome has been synthesised, and integrated with the help of integrase into the genome of the target cell as a provirus (**Figure 2**) (Willet & Hoise, 2013).(Willet & Hoise, 2013)When the cell with the integrated provirus divides, the daughter cells receive the DNA of the integrated virus, causing the infection to remain constant and can only be eliminated if all cells with the provirus are destroyed. This makes therapy against FeLV infections very complicated, as it not only has to be aimed at restricting the formation of infectious viral particles and preventing new infections, but also at destroying the already infected cells. (Palmero & Carballés Pérez, 2010) (Collado A, 2017).

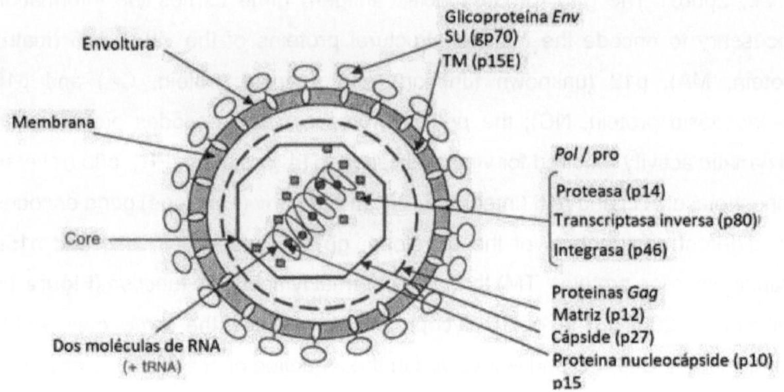

Figure 1. Structure of FeLV. *Env* encodes surface and transmembrane glycoproteins, *gag* and *pro* genes encode capsid and protease proteins, respectively. Modified from (Poulet et al., 2003)..

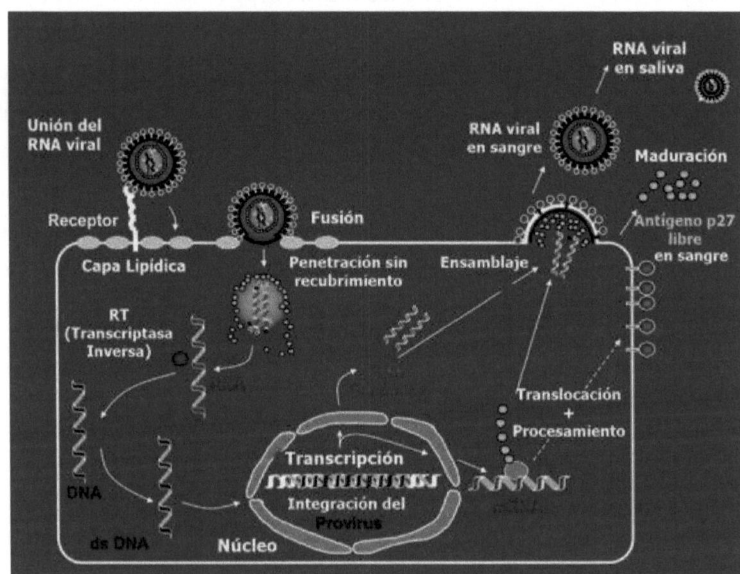

Figure 2. FeLV replication. Once FeLV has bound and fused with the host cell, the viral RNA is released and converted into viral DNA. The viral DNA is transferred to the cell nucleus during cell division, where it is integrated into the host genomic DNA with the help of an integrase and is then called proviral DNA. When the cell becomes active, new viral RNAs and proteins are produced and assemble on the host cell membrane to build new viral particles that are shed into the blood and saliva. In addition to viral particles, the soluble FeLV p27 capsid antigen is also excreted into the blood and can be detected by laboratory ELISA and rapid tests (Hartmann & Hofmann-Lehmann, 2020)..

6.4. FeLV GENETIC DIVERSITY

There are two forms of FeLV, the endogenous (enFeLV) which does not cause disease but is relevant to FeLV biology (Chiu et al., 2018). (Chiu et al., 2018); and the exogenous form (exFeLV) which has 5 subgroups: A, B, C, D and T with different receptors. FeLV-A is the most abundant transmissible form and two subtypes were created from it, as its recombination with an endogenous domestic cat virus resulted in FeLV-B, and mutations that accumulated in the *env* gene of FeLV-A led to the emergence of FeLV-C (Guliukina et al., 2019).. FeLV-T is a chimeric virus resulting from the recombination between viruses 61E and 61C (Chiu et al., 2018).

6.4.1. ENDOGENIC FORM OF FeLV

Retroviruses require integration of their genome into the host chromosome to complete their cycle, this provirus in the genome is not passed on to the offspring. (López-Goñi, 2015)However, if the retrovirus infects a germ cell, the provirus can be inherited as a cellular gene and be present in the genome of the offspring, if the gamete carries the DNA of the virus, after fertilisation all the cells of the new embryo will carry the provirus in their genome. This has been happening for millions of years in many organisms, and is called Endogenous RetroVirus (ERV), which have become "fossilised" in the genome. This is a "vertical" transfer of the virus, from parent to offspring, which allows the "fixation" of these ERVs in the population. (Feschotte & Gilbert, 2012)..

In the *Felis* genus, enFeLVs, which are a replica of the defective provirus, are 86% similar to exFeLV at the nucleotide level and the differences between them are in *gag* and *env*, insertions and deletions (INDELs[1]), frameshifts, nonsense mutations and changes in the regions, mutations and changes in the unique 3' regions of the LTR, as shown in **Figure** 3 (Chiu et al., 2018). Proviral DNA expression is restricted to subgenomic transcripts[2] that prevent assembly of the infectious virus. However, enFeLV DNA fragments can recombine with exogenous FeLV resulting in recombinant viruses, as in the case of FeLV-B. It has been suggested that enFeLVs might be involved in exogenous retroviral infection, either by suppressing exogenous virus replication or by enhancing exogenous viral infection (Guliukina et al., 2019)..

6.4.2. EXOGENOUS FORM OF FeLV

It is horizontally transmitted, can replicate and has the 5 main subgroups, and as briefly explained in the "FeLV genetic diversity" topic, the subgroups arise during virus replication due to errors during transcription and recombination with FeLVs in the genome; the subgroups are distinguished genetically by differences in the *env* gene and functionally by interaction with different host cell receptors for entry (**Table 1**). (Ahmad & Levy, 2010).

---

[1] "Indel" is a general term that can refer to the insertion, deletion or insertion and deletion of nucleotides in genomic DNA. Some types of DNA alterations, including insertions/deletions (indels), are not necessarily the direct result of DNA damage, *per se*. Instead, indels can originate from DNA polymerase errors or from improper DNA repair after genetic damage. Sehn, J. K. (2015). Insertions and deletions (Indels). In S. Kulkarni & J. Pfeifer (Eds.), *Clinical Genomics* (1st ed., pp. 130-148). Academic Press. .

[2] These are fragments of the genome that, while lacking some of the information contained in the virus' RNA, retain all the genes necessary for self-replication, i.e. those for proteins and those for the virus' own genomic elements that are necessary for replication and translation. In this way, they are able to produce new subgenomic molecules which, in turn, can continue to replicate, although they are not able to give rise to complete infectious viruses. Puig-Basagoti, F., & Saíz, J. C. (2001). Subgenomic replicons of hepatitis C virus (HCV): new expectations for hepatitis C prophylaxis and treatment. *Gastroenterology and Hepatology*, *24*(10), 506-510.

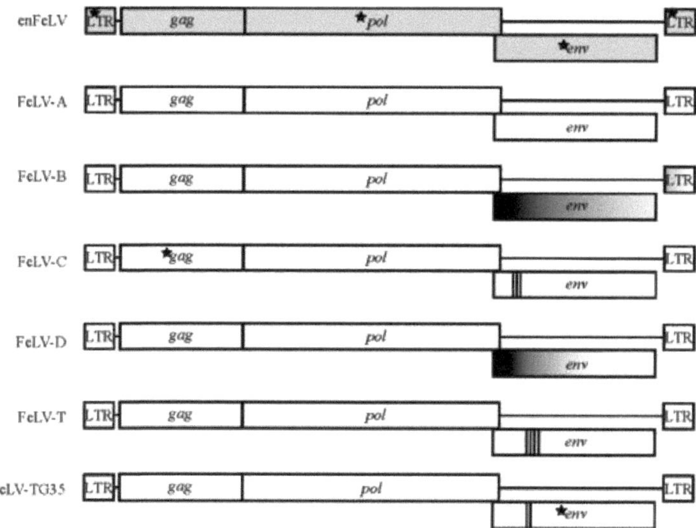

Figure 3. Genomic map of FeLV subgroups. Six different FeLV subgroups have been associated with different disease outcomes that differ genetically and biologically from endogenous FeLV (enFeLV). The enFeLV is the most genetically distinct from FeLV-A, with nucleotide differences observed in the long terminal repeats (LTR), the gag and *env*. FeLV-B is formed by recombination of the enFeLV *env-LTR* with FeLV-A. The 5' recombination site is more conserved than the 3' site. FeLV-C, T, and TG35 have focal insertions, substitutions and deletions within the FeLV-A virus of origin in different regions. Insertions are most often located in the 5' *env* and are demarcated here by bold vertical bars, with each line denoting a minimum of one amino acid insertion. Stars denote the presence of single nucleotide polymorphisms (SNPs) that are highly concentrated in the respective genes between FeLV-A and other subgroups. FeLV-D shows a recombination event with another endogenous domestic cat virus (Chiu et al., 2018).

Table 1. Specific receptors for the different FeLV subgroups. (Guliukina et al., 2019)

FeLV subgroups	Cellular Receiver	Receiver function
FeLV-A	THTR1	Thiamine transporter protein
FeLV-B	Fe-Pit1 and Fe-Pit2	NA-dependent inorganic phosphate transporter
FeLV-C	FLVCR	Heme transporter protein[3]
FeLV-T	Fe-Pit1	NA-dependent inorganic phosphate transporter

6.4.2.1. SUB-GROUP A

It is the most abundant subgroup and the only one that spreads horizontally in nature and is a helper for the other subgroups, as cats infected with subgroup B and C are co-infected with A; for this reason vaccines only protect against it. It has been reported to be the least pathogenic and has been associated with macrocytic anaemia, immunosuppression and thymic lymphoma of T-cell origin (Chiu et al., 2018; Guliukina et al., 2019; Levy, 2008; Willet & Hoise, 2013)..

6.4.2.2. SUB- GROUP B

A recombinant DNA proviral of FeLV-A and enFeLV, FeLV-A occurs in nearly 50% of cats and is the most morbid and lethal due to the development of leukaemia and lymphoma, is tumourigenic and is only transmitted with FeLV-A (Chiu et al., 2018; Guliukina et al., 2019; Hartman & Sykes, 2014)..

6.4.2.3. SUB-GROUP C

FeLV-C virus has emerged as a result of multiple mutations in the *env* gene (SU) of FeLV-A virus, this subgroup has been associated with the development of aplastic anaemia (Chiu et al., 2018; Guliukina et al., 2019)..

---

[3] A metal complex of ferrous ion and porphyrin; component of haemoglobin and some other biologically important haemoproteins.

6.4.2.4. SUB-GROUP T

FeLV-61C, or FeLV-T, can induce persistent viraemia and feline acquired immunodeficiency syndrome (FAID), named by Gasper et al. in 1987, after isolating a type of FeLV that was intensely immunosuppressive (Gasper et al., 1987). (Gasper et al., 1987)was characterised after experimental infections of a domestic cat with a transmissible FeLV clone 61E, also an infected cat developed a thymic lymphoma and sequence analysis revealed a primary envelope variant of FeLV-A (Chiu et al., 2018). To infect T lymphocytes, FeLV-T expresses on its viral envelope a membrane glycoprotein that binds to and attaches to a target cell receptor molecule (Fe-Pit1) (Hartman & Sykes, 2014).

6.4.2.5. NEW SUB-GROUPS

There are two new variants that are less abundant, FeLV-D and TG35. FeLV-D was identified simultaneously with the discovery of a new endogenous domestic cat retrovirus (ERV-DC). Insertion of the ERV-DC *env* gene into FeLV would result in the emergence of FeLV-D, and was identified in four cats, three of which, had haematopoietic tumours (Chiu et al., 2018). It is theorised that its replication is regulated by the antiretroviral factor "restriction for feline retrovirus X (Refrex-1)", however the mechanism by which this takes place is still unclear, but it is suggested that Refrex-1 has is important in restricting viral replication and protecting felines, as it is thought to compete with FeLV-D for cellular receptors, preventing the virus from penetrating (Chiu et al., 2018; Guliukina et al., 2019)..

6.5. TRANSMISSION

FeLV is transmitted horizontally, mainly via saliva between infected cats and susceptible cats with close contact, so during affiliative social behaviour or fighting, a healthy cat may come into contact with the virus, it is also possible for transmission to occur when they sneeze and share the same litter or litter box and food bowls, however the viral envelope is soluble in lipids, disinfectants, soap, heat and drying, so FeLV is inactivated in the environment in a matter of minutes. The virus can also be spread in urine and faeces at lower concentrations, as FeLV is present in various tissues, body fluids and secretions, but this is less common. Venereal transmission is also possible, as virus and infected cells have been isolated in semen, vaginal fluid and urogenital epithelium. Fleas have been considered as a route of transmission, as viral RNA has been detected in fleas and faeces, but it appears that fleas do not play an important role in transmission in nature. Iatrogenic transmission may occur via contaminated needles, instruments or blood transfusions. Regressively infected cats do not shed the virus via saliva and other excretions, but blood transfusions from regressively infected cats have been shown to effectively transmit the virus, thus infecting recipient cats (Hartmann, 2012b; Hartmann, 2012b; Hartmann, 2012b; Hartmann, 2012b; Hartmann, 2012b; Hartmann, 2012b; Hartmann, 2012b; Hartmann, 2012b; Hartmann, 2012b; Hartmann, 2012b). (Hartmann, 2012b; Hartmann & Hofmann-Lehmann, 2020; Heredia, 2019)

FeLV is a widely distributed pathogen in domestic cats and domestic cats have a wide distribution in different habitats, so it is not uncommon for FeLV to jump to other genera, infecting the Florida Panther (*Puma concolor*) (Brown et al., 2008)the Iberian lynx (*Lynx pardinus*) in Spain (Luaces et al., 2008) and captive-born jaguarundi (*Puma yagouaroundi*) (Willet & Hoise, 2013)

This is of interest because of the impact on this population, although there are not many reports mentioning the presence of endogenous retroviruses and their implications. Autran et *al* (2016) reported the presence of endogenous retroviruses in domestic cats suggesting a regulatory or protective function in PCR-positive cats. Recently, Garcia-Ortiz (MSc Thesis, data in progress, 2024) found that FeLV viral load detected by quantitative PCR in cats with different stages of disease correlated with disease progression and prognosis, however, final results of phylogenetic analysis are required to corroborate this information. (Ramirez et al., 2016)..

Viremic females can transmit the infection vertically to the offspring, becoming infected via the transplacental route, when the mother licks the offspring or via colostrum. Transmission also occurs in cats with regressive infection or atypical focal infection, because the infection can be reactivated during gestation. If infection occurs in utero, fetal resorption, abortion and neonatal death are common, however, 20% of vertically infected kittens are born and subsequently become persistently infected adults, it has also been observed that these newborn kittens have negative antigen test results at birth, but may test positive in the following weeks or months once the virus begins to replicate. (Hartmann, 2012b; Hartmann & Hofmann-Lehmann, 2020)..

6.6. COURSE OF INFECTION

FeLV infection has been documented to have different stages, as diagnostic tools such as PCR have provided new insights into the course of infection. It was found that, if a cat has been infected it does not become immune, as the FeLV provirus is integrated into the host genome, it is unlikely to be completely eliminated after infection, and remains provirus positive. Cats that are antigenemia negative[4] and provirus positive are considered carriers and do not shed the virus, however, it is possible for the virus to reactivate and exhibit recurrent shedding. Based on this information, a new classification was proposed, in which the stages of FeLV infection are defined as abortive infection (formerly 'regressor cats'), regressive infection (formerly 'transient viraemia' followed by 'latent infection'), progressive infection (formerly 'persistent viraemia') and focal or atypical infection, see **Table 2 and Figure** 4 (Hartmann, 2012a) Knowledge of the different courses of infection is relevant for the interpretation of diagnostic test results and the application of appropriate therapeutic and epidemiological measures, about diagnostic methods I will discuss below.

Table 2. Stages of feline leukaemia virus (FeLV) infection. Modified from (Hartmann, 2012a).

Stages of FeLV infection	Blood p27 antigen	Viral isolation from blood	Viral RNA in blood	Viral DNA in blood	Viral isolation from tissue	Dissemin ation of the virus	FeLV-associated diseases
Focal	Variabl e	Variable	Variab le	Variab le	Variable	Variable	Unlikely
Abortifacie nt	Negati ve	Negative	Negati ve	Negati ve	Negative	Negative	Unlikely

[4] Presence of soluble viral capsid protein p27 in blood; in most cats this is considered equivalent to viraemia (Little et al., 2020).

Regressive	Negative	Negative	Negative	Positive	Negative	Negative	Unlikely
Progressive	Positive	Positive	Positive	Positive	Positive	Positive	Likely

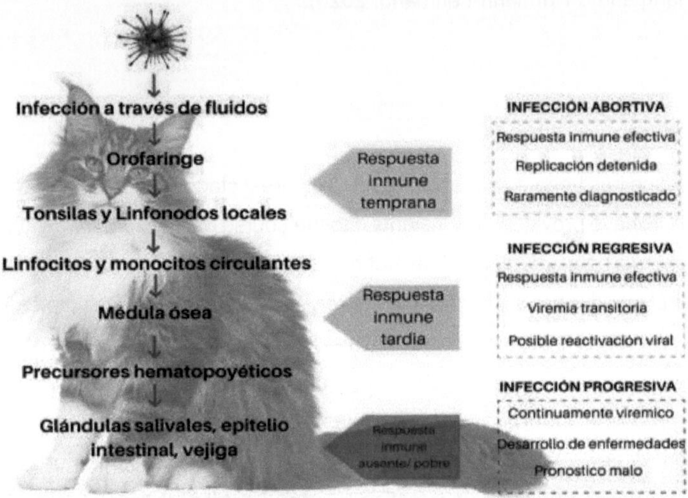

Figure 4. Exposure outcomes are largely influenced by the immune response to infection. Abortive infection is the result of a low dose of FeLV exposure or an effective and specific immune response early in the infection. Regressive infection is the result of an effective immune response later in the infection, either just before or just after bone marrow infiltration. Cats with regressive infection are transiently antigenic and viremic. After weeks or months, viraemia is controlled and these cats become "non-viremic". Progressive infection is the result of a poor immune response. Progressively infected cats are continuously viraemic and have a poor prognosis, developing FeLV-associated disease and often have a limited lifespan. (Yasmin et al., 2021)..

Cats with **progressive infection** are infected in the bone marrow, resulting in persistent viraemia, where granulocytes, platelets, lymphocytes and monocytes in the peripheral blood are infected with the virus. This infection is characterised by persistent viraemia/antigenemia that is not effectively controlled at onset and an absence of FeLV-specific immune response, so that the virus infects permanently and the cat remains infectious, they have persistent viraemia, p27 antigen is found in blood and they have neither virus-neutralising antibodies nor high levels of FeLV-specific cytotoxic lymphocytes. They usually develop life-threatening FeLV-associated disease sometimes within months, however many of these cats with proper care can have a quality of life and live for many years, it is estimated that at least 30% of FeLV-exposed cats develop progressive infection and virus-associated disease, and 60% develop an effective and long-lasting immune response leading to regressive infection. (Hofmann-Lehmann & Hartmann, 2020; Hoover et al., 2005; Murphy, 2016)..

Regressive infection develops due to an effective immune response where the cat has recovered from the primary viraemia and viral replication was contained before or shortly after bone marrow infection, these cats also do not usually develop FeLV-related disease. (Hartmann, 2012a; Hofmann-Lehmann & Hartmann, 2020).. The disappearance of viraemia is due to an effective immune response, where cats produce neutralising antibodies and FeLV-specific cytotoxic T lymphocytes (CTL), which is believed to be essential for immunity, as infected cells are eliminated by CTL activity (Argyl et al., 2001). (Argyl et al., 2001). Clearance of antigenemia can be observed within 1 to 12 weeks, up to 40 weeks, and in rare cases can take months, but the likelihood of clearance of viraemia decreases with time. Most cats with regressive infection do not develop bone marrow infection, so occasionally lymphocytes and monocytes are provirus positive and it is uncommon to detect viral RNA in peripheral blood, however, as noted above the likelihood of clearance of viraemia decreases with time, there are reports that if viraemia persists for more than three weeks the bone marrow is at risk of becoming infected and with it the haematopoietic precursors, so infected granulocytes and platelets may circulate in the body, but a small percentage of these cats are able to clear the viraemia without completely eliminating the virus, Highly sensitive PCR assays demonstrate the presence of provirus in blood leukocytes and tissues, and has been termed "latent infection" which is defined by the presence of provirus in the genome without production of virus protein, because during cell division proviral DNA is replicated and the information is given to daughter cells, Therefore, entire cell lineages may contain proviral DNA, but the proviral DNA is not translated into protein and no infectious viral particles are produced, so that cats with regressive infection are not infectious and usually test negative for FeLV antigen; However, as the proviral DNA is still present in the cat's cells, there is a risk of reactivation if immunosuppression is present, as the immune system only keeps the virus under control and does not eliminate it completely, so if it is not able to suppress viral replication and viraemia recurs, the cat may excrete the virus and develop FeLV-associated diseases (Hartmann, 2012a; Hofmann-Lehmann & Hartmann, 2020; Murphy, 2016)..

Abortive infection occurs when a cat has a low level of exposure to the virus, e.g. in indirect transmission with contaminated faeces, and has strong anti-FeLV immunity, these cats can avoid viral replication by effective humoral and cellular responses and have high levels of neutralising antibodies, so they never become viraemic. (Hartmann, 2012a; Hofmann-Lehmann & Hartmann, 2020)..

During **focal or atypical infection** cats are p27 antigen positive, but there is no isolation of infectious virus, so these cats are antigenaemic with an absence of replicating virus, this condition can persist for years as the cat's immune system keeps virus replication retained in tissues such as the spleen, lymph nodes, small intestine, urinary tract, eyes or mammary gland. This infection can give confusing results in FeLV tests, as it can alternate negative and positive results, and has been reported in up to 10% of naturally infected cats, there is a case of a female cat that tested negative for p27 antigen, however, the virus was retained in mammary gland and transmitted the virus to kittens via milk (Cattori et al., 2007b; Hartmann, 2012a; Hofmann-Lehmann & Hartmann, 2020; Murphy, 2016)..

The variety of courses of infection shows that there are differences in the way cats respond immunologically to FeLV.

6.7. IMMUNE RESPONSE TO FeLV VIRUS

Host control of viral infections involves both innate and adaptive responses. The former is mediated primarily by type I interferons (IFN-I), macrophages/monocytes and NK cell responses. The adaptive immune response is mediated by T and B cells, after the primary infection has resolved, thus developing the long-lasting component of immunological memory, i.e. antibody production. The magnitude and quality of the innate immune response is intimately involved in the subsequent primary adaptive response, which in turn determines the magnitude and quality of the memory response. (Alsharifi et al., 2008)..

Immunity is an important determinant of the outcome of FeLV infections in cats. (Jarret & Russell, 1978). Although outcome depends primarily on the immune and age status of the cat, it is also affected by the pathogenicity of the virus, the pressure of infection and the concentration of virus. The outcome of infection by also depends on the genetic variation of the virus and the cat population in which it naturally occurs. FeLV strains were shown to increase the efficiency of receptor binding, longitudinal studies[5] showed certain mutations leading to faster disease onset and substitutions in certain genes altered the outcome of infection, suggesting that different LTR and surface (SU) genes are involved in pathogenesis (Hartman & Sykes, 2014).

Host interaction with the virus during the first 4 weeks may result in either **a)** the inability of the host immune response to contain viral replication in lymphonodes, epithelia and bone marrow precursor cells or **b)** a successful immune response resulting in reduced viral replication **(Hoover et al., 2005)**. (Hoover et al., 2005)..

Retroviral infections alter defence mechanisms, allowing secondary infections to occur. To our knowledge, there are four mechanisms by which FeLV can cause immunopathological disease. First, FeLV infects rapidly dividing cells (thymus, lymph nodes, spleen, bone marrow and macrophages), resulting in decreased cell numbers due to their destruction, or FeLV alters their function (the envelope protein p15) has been shown to abrogate feline lymphocyte blastogenesis in *vitro*. Secondly, antibody reaction to membrane antigens on lymphocytes, neutrophils and macrophages. Thirdly, persistently infected cats have a continuous supply of FeLV antigens, so that the formation of immune antibodies would lead to the development of disease due to FeLV antigens. Finally, FeLV-induced

[5] The longitudinal study implies the existence of repeated measures (more than two) over a follow-up period. It would therefore be a subtype of a cohort study (group of individuals who share a common characteristic) that allows inferences to be drawn at the individual level and allows changes in different variables (exposures and effects) and transitions between different health states to be analysed. Delgado Rodríguez, M., & Llorca Díaz, J. (2004). Longitudinal studies: concept and particularities. *Revista Española de Salud Pública*, *78*(2), 141-148.

transformation results in the expression of FOCMA on the membrane of transformed lymphocytes and, if FOCMA antibody is produced, these cells can be lysed and cause lymphopenia (Hardy, 1982). (Hardy, 1982)..

6.7.1. INNATE IMMUNITY

The initial immune response plays an essential role in determining the outcome of viral infection, however the cat's innate antiviral immune system remains poorly understood, so it is still unclear what the initial response to infection looks like and how it might be manipulated in favour of the host (Cattori et al., 2011)..

Innate immunity encompasses defence mechanisms that are non-specific, spontaneous and without memory. These could be grouped into tissue (skin and mucous membranes), cellular (inflammation, phagocytosis, cellular cytotoxicity) and molecular (complement, interferon, acute phase proteins, etc.). (Montaraz C, 2012).

6.7.1.1. INTEGUMENTARY SYSTEM

The virus is ingested or inhaled and is deposited in the mucosa of the oral and nasal pharynx (tonsils), attaches, infects and replicates locally in mucosal epithelial cells, mucosa-associated lymphocytes and macrophages (MALT), it is not yet known how the virus penetrates the mucus layer to gain access to mucosal epithelial cells or whether mucosal macrophages and/or dendritic cells are involved in the infection. Virus subgroups use envelope glycoproteins, probably surface glycoprotein (SU) and transmembrane protein (TM), to attach to receptors and enter T lymphocytes, other lymphocytes, and mucosal epithelial cells (Horzinek, 1988; Horzinek, 1988; Horzinek, 1988; Horzinek, 1988; Horzinek, 1988; Horzinek, 1988). (Horzinek, 1988; Zachary, 2017)..

Infected cells spread by trafficking leukocytes and macrophages through lymphatic vessels to regional pharyngeal lymphocytes, where it replicates and infects other lymphocytes and macrophages. B lymphocytes are suspected to be the primary cells used to spread the virus by trafficking leukocytes, while T lymphocytes appear to be the main target cell for infection. Once regional lymph nodes are infected, the virus spreads in B lymphocytes by leukocyte trafficking to the circulatory system, via postcapillary veins or lymphatic vessels and the thoracic duct to lymph nodes and lymphoid organs, such as the spleen and Peyer's patches. FeLV replicates in rapidly dividing cells such as intestinal endothelial crypt cells and germinal centre B cells, and if the immune response does not intervene after initial infection, FeLV spreads to epithelial and glandular tissues throughout the body, which typically include salivary, tonsillar, pharyngeal, bladder, gastric, intestinal, pancreatic, endometrial and endothelial tissue, spreading to bone marrow and infecting haematopoietic precursor cells (**Figure 5**), once haematological and immune stem cells are infected, viral clearance is impossible (Hardy, 1982; Hause, 1982; Hause, 1982). (Hardy, 1982; Hause et al., 1979; Zachary, 2017)..

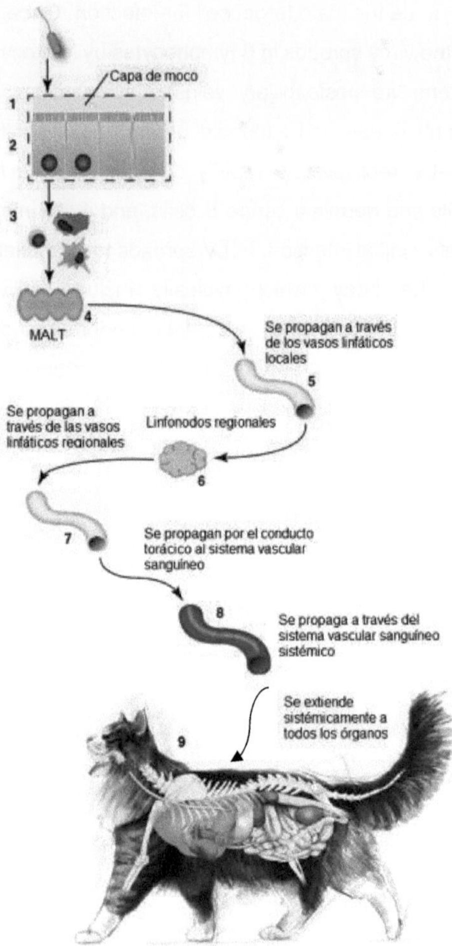

Figure 5. The spread of FeLV to organs. 1) FeLV must penetrate the mucosal epithelium. 2) FeLV crosses mucosal, serosal or integumentary barriers. 3) FeLV encounters mucosa-associated cells (e.g. lymphocytes, macrophages and dendritic cells). 4) It spreads locally to lymphoid tissues (e.g. mucosa-associated lymphoid tissue [MALT] such as tonsils). 5) FeLV spreads regionally in afferent lymphatic vessels. 6) FeLV encounters cells in regional lymph nodes. 7) FeLV spreads systemically in efferent lymphatic vessels to the thoracic duct and anterior vena cava. 8) FeLV spreads systemically in the circulatory system. 9) FeLV spreads to lymphoid organs, such as the spleen and Peyer's patches, and then the mucous membranes of the salivary glands or bone marrow, as modified from (Zachary, 2017).

6.7.1.2. DIGESTIVE TRACT

FeLV has been associated with alimentary lymphoma which is common in cats over 8 years of age, arising from B cells of the lamina propria in any part of the gastrointestinal tract or mesenteric lymph nodes, clinical signs are usually palpable tumours and gastroenteric signs such as vomiting, diarrhoea or constipation, and weight loss. (Cotter, 1992; Essex et al., 1981; Hardy, 1981)..

In addition to alimentary lymphoma, "Feline panleukopenia-like syndrome (FPLS)" or "FeLV-associated enteritis (FAE)" has also been described. Erosion of the small intestinal villi has been reported resulting in diarrhoea, vomiting and anorexia, giving opportunity for secondary infections and other signs such as oral ulceration or gingivitis; during infection FeLV pg70 and p15E proteins were found in the epithelial cells of the intestinal crypt (**Fig. 6, 7 and 8**), suggesting that this is the cause of the development of enteric signology, it has also been described that the intestinal mucosal infiltration is dominated by T-lymphocytes, mainly $CD8^+$, pointing to a local cytotoxic T-cell response in the FAE. Other findings include aplastic bone marrow with reduced granulocytes resulting in neutropenia, lymphoid depletion, haemorrhagic necrosis of mesenteric, cecal, colonic and sublumbar lymph nodes, however, other authors mention that the lymphoid tissues are unchanged or even hyperplastic as cats showing no change in enterocytes have been observed to have variable lymphoid tissue activity and a tendency for increased bone marrow activity, as in some cats with FAE, bone marrow activity was normal and lymphoid tissue was unchanged or hyperplastic, this has also been observed in early stages of experimental infection with FeLV-FAIDS variants, which is thought to be the cause of FAE, however, although viral replication can be observed in lymphoid tissues of cats with FeLV-FAIDS and FAE, there is still no evidence that FeLV has a cytopathic effect on lymphoid and haematopoietic cells (Grant et al., 2000; Grant et al., 2000; Grant et al., 2000). (Grant et al., 2000; Hardy, 1982; Hartmann, 2012a; Jackson et al., 2001; Reinacher, 1989)..

Immunofluorescence and electron microscopy have shown feline panleukopenia virus (FPV) antigen in the intestine of cats that died after being infected with FeLV despite being negative for FPV antigen, so it is unclear whether the syndrome could be caused by co-infection with FPV or by FeLV itself, as during other studies where cats were experimentally infected with FeLV-FAIDS, proliferation of FeLV antigen within enterocytes was observed, causing FAE-like signology, suggesting that development of FPLS and/or FAE may be dependent on FeLV strain (Hartmann, 2012a; Hartmann, 2014)..

Figure 6. FAE in jejunum. a. Moderate alterations in epithelial cells, degeneration of intestinal crypt epithelial cells (arrow). Moderate mononuclear infiltration of the mucosa. **b.** Severe alterations of the crypt epithelial cells. Crypts have flattened epithelium and degenerated intraluminal cells. Moderate mononuclear infiltration of the mucosa. (Grant et al., 2000).

a. **b.**

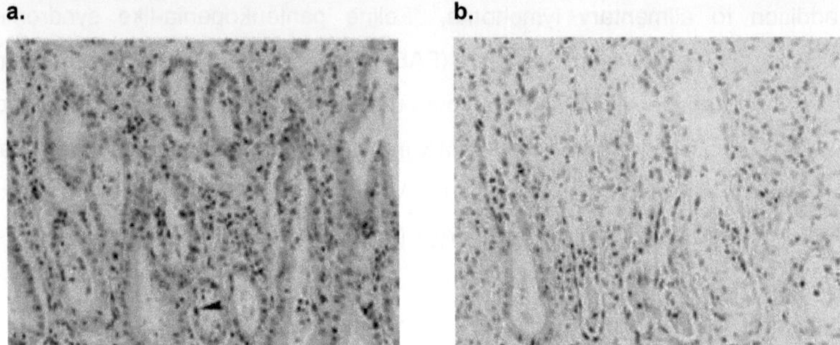

Figure 7. FAE cat jejunum, Expression of FeLV antigens in epithelial cells. a. Cytoplasmic staining of many crypt epithelial cells for gp70. Isolated infiltrating cells in the mucosa (arrow). b. Moderate cytoplasmic staining of many epithelial cells in the crypt for p27 (Grant et al., 2000).

a. **b.** **c.**

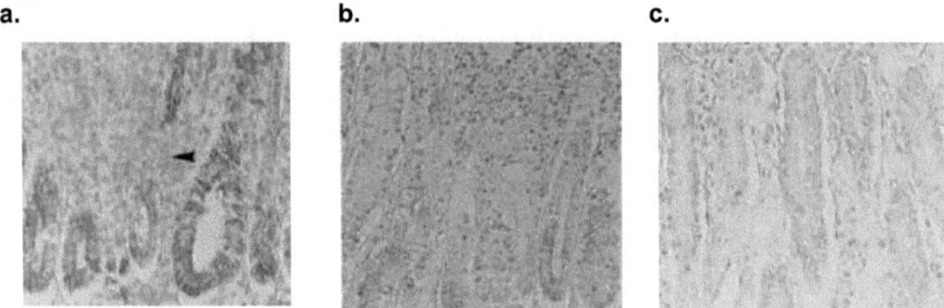

Figure 8. FeLV-positive cat without intestinal alterations. a. Mild to moderate cytoplasmic staining of numerous crypt epithelial cells for gp70. **b.** Crypt epithelial cells and mucosal infiltrating cells are p15E-negative. **c.** Strongly positive cytoplasmic staining of many crypt epithelial cells for p70. (Grant et al., 2000).

a. **b.** **c.**

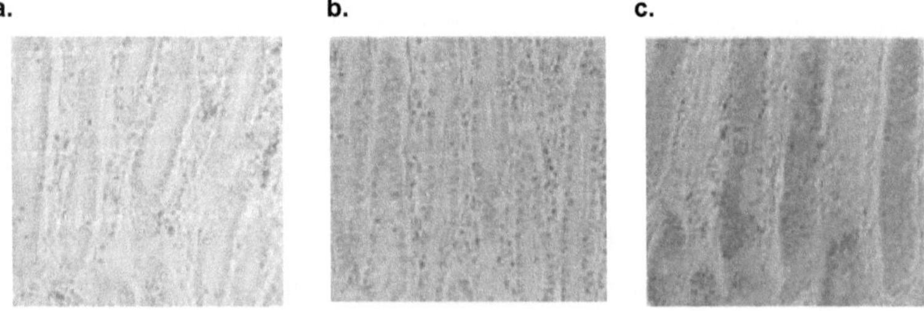

6.7.1.3. RESPIRATORY TRACT

It is well known that FeLV positive cats are susceptible to secondary diseases due to immunosuppression, inflammatory respiratory tract diseases such as rhinitis, feline influenza, pneumonia or pleuritis have been reported in 10% of cats with persistent FeLV, another documented disease is sporotrichosis caused by the fungus *S. schenckii*, in one study 22% of 142 cats tested were co-infected, sporotrichosis usually causes respiratory signs and skin lesions (Reinacher, 1989; Schubach et al., 2004). (Reinacher, 1989; Schubach et al., 2004)..

Nasal or nasopharyngeal lymphomas are uncommon and usually account for 1% of all feline tumours, but are commonly seen in male cats, as due to their territorial behaviour it is believed that FeLV transmission may be more efficient. In general, this type of lymphoma usually originates in the upper respiratory tract (URT), mostly in the nose, 10% in the nasopharynx and 8% in both anatomical sites. In a study in which 164 biopsies of TRS lymphomas were performed, p27 and gp70 antigen were detected in 21 lymphomas (Avallone et al., 2006; Avallone et al., 2006). (Avallone et al., 2015).. Mediastinal lymphoma has also been reported in young FeLV-positive cats, presenting with dyspnoea, cough or regurgitation, due to enlarged mediastinal lymph nodes, the prognosis of these cats is poor and they usually live for 3 to 4 months (Couto, 2000)..

Another uncommon type of tumour described in the nasal cavity is the spontaneous feline olfactory neuroblastoma, which originates in the neuroectoderm, it is a very invasive and highly metastatic tumour, the clinical signs in addition to nasal discharge and sneezing can be neurological, This may be due to the tumour invading the central nervous system (CNS), FeLV particles have been found in these tumours, suggesting that the virus may cause it (Higgins et al., 1990). (Higgins et al., 1990; Malinowski, 2006)..

6.7.1.4. REPRODUCTIVE TRACT

There are reports of FeLV transmission via urine, milk, semen, vaginal fluids and placenta. (Palmero & Carballés Pérez, 2010).. An infected mother can transmit the virus to the foetus or newborn via transplacental and colostrum, FeLV has been shown experimentally to cause foetal death, resorption, placental involution and second trimester abortion, and although the mechanism by which FeLV causes foetal death is still unknown, a similar syndrome has been described in female mice infected with murine viral leukaemia (MuLV), which causes foetal death as the MuLV provirus inserts itself into the alpha collagen gene of embryos and prevents collagen synthesis, causing blood vessels and connective tissues to weaken leading to fatal haemorrhage, so FeLV could cause foetal death by a similar pattern (Hardy, 1993). (Hardy, 1993)..

Cats have an endotheliochorial placenta which is a barrier that prevents the passage of maternal immunoglobulins to the fetus, thus 5-10% of maternally derived antibodies (MDA) are transmitted during gestation to fetuses, however, FeLV replication has been observed in fetal haematopoietic cells and not in the placenta, suggesting that the maternal anti-FeLV response did not stop the passage of the virus (Frymus, 2017; Rojko et al., 1982; Schultz et al., 1974; Scott et al., 1970)..

Cats with regressive infection may have live kittens even after aborting previous litters, but these kittens will have congenital or perinatal FeLV infections, (Hardy, 1993). In latently infected cats (ELISA negative) the virus may reactivate during gestation and become infectious, or the virus may remain exclusively in the mammary gland (focal infection) and kittens will be infected through lactation (Palmero & Carballés Pérez, 1993). (Palmero & Carballés Pérez, 2010)..

Although FeLV has not been documented, during FIV infection the virus has been isolated in vaginal swabs from pregnant females, kittens born to these females have had the virus at birth and others 6 months later, so it is theorised that the latter were infected at the end of gestation or during delivery, something similar is believed to occur with FeLV (O'Neil et al., 1996)..

FeLV has been isolated from semen of acutely and chronically infected cats, so females could become infected after being inseminated laparoscopically, however it is unknown how often free-living cats can become infected via seminal route, but it is believed to be low (Hartmann, 2012b; Heredia, 2019). (Hartmann, 2012b; Heredia, 2019)..

6.7.1.5. PHYSICAL AND CHEMICAL FACTORS

6.7.1.5.1. SKIN

FeLV can cause skin tumours such as lymphomas and fibrosarcomas, and other clinical signs such as pyoderma, dermatophytosis, demodicosis and Malassezia dermatitis, as well as poor wound healing, seborrhoea and generalised pruritus; FeLV has also been associated with two different skin syndromes, cutaneous horns (**Fig. 9**) and giant cell dermatosis; cutaneous horns are a benign hyperplasia of keratinocytes that has been described in cats with FeLV (Favrot et al., 2005; Hartmann, 2012a; Nagata & Rosenkrantz, 2013)..

In general, squamous cell dermatosis may cause crusting, alopecia, itching in the face and neck area or other signs such as vesicular and ulcerative lesions on the pads and mucous membranes or other parts of the body (**Fig. 10**), which do not respond to treatment with antibiotics and corticosteroids, have a poor prognosis and usually die days or weeks after onset; they are negative on scrapings for parasites and fungi, but are ELISA positive and immunohistochemical analysis of dermal lesions shows epithelial cells, hair follicles, sebaceous glands and lymphocytes in dermal infiltrates expressing viral proteins (**Fig. 11**); on histology, ulcerative dermatitis with folliculitis, dyskeratotic keratinocytes and the formation of syncytia within the epidermis and sebaceous glands can be observed (**Fig.12 and 13**), formation of syncytial-type giant cells with up to 30 nuclei and abundant cytoplasm; thus necrotic lesions of erosion and ulceration are the result of loss of epidermal integrity caused by giant cell formation and dyskeratosis. FeLV variants have been shown to exhibit diverse pathogenic and cytopathic effects, so it is possible that FeLV-induced giant cell dermatosis may be the result of a specific and probably rare viral variant (Favrot et al., 2005; Gross et al., 1993)..

Cutaneous lymphomas in cats are rare and usually occur in older cats with negative FeLV serology, but recently viral genome and antigens have been demonstrated in the neoplastic cells of this type of lymphoma suggesting a focal infection, immunohistochemistry is not routinely performed in these tumours so it is unknown how often FeLV might be the cause. (Favrot et al., 2005).

Figure 10. Cutaneous horns. a. in the dorsolumbar area of a cat. (Rees & Goldschmidt, 1998) and in **b.** palmar pads of a Persian cat (Souza et al., 2010).

a. **b.**

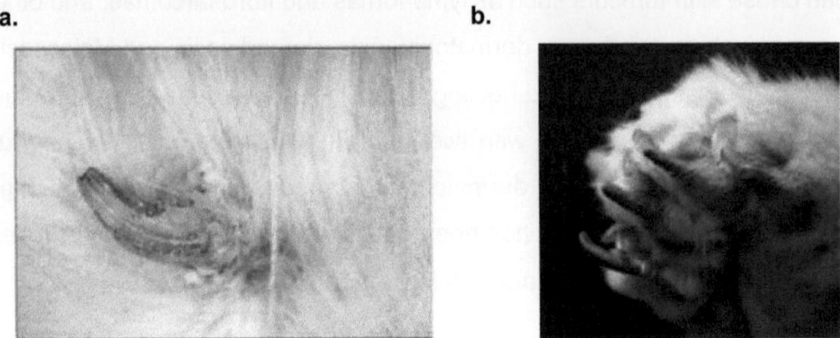

Figure 11. Ulcerative lesions. a. Facial lesion of cat ELISA (+) to FeLV and **b.** carpal lesion of cat ELISA (-) to FeLV, but immunohistochemistry showed expression of viral proteins (Favrot et al., **2005**). (Favrot et al., 2005).

a. **b.**

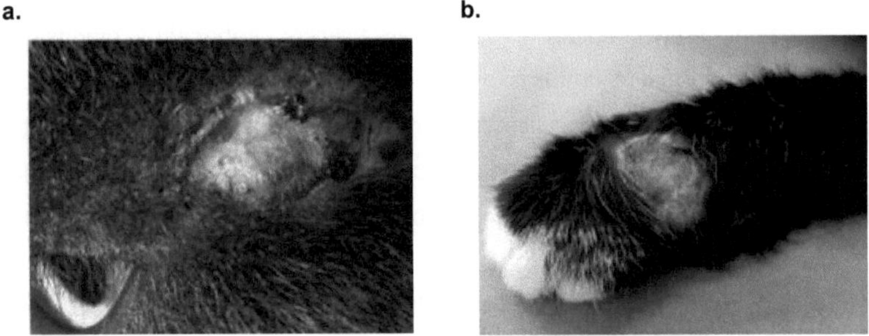

Figure 12. Immunohistochemistry. a. Epithelial cells expressing FeLV gp70 antigen (arrows). **b.** Neoplastic cells (arrowhead) and epidermal keratinocytes (arrow) expressing FeLV antigens (Favrot et al., 2005). (Favrot et al., 2005).

a.

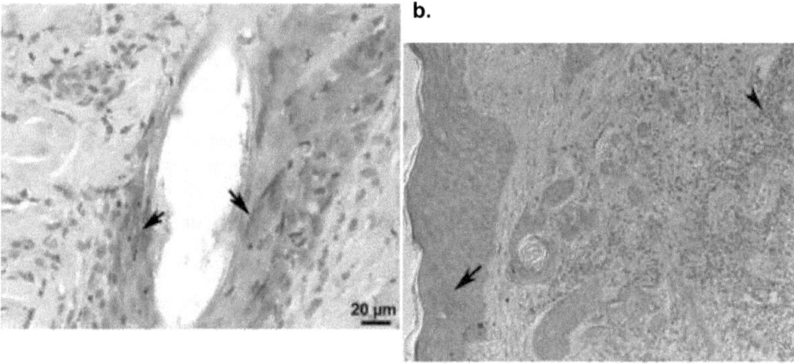

Figure 13. Histology of skin lesions. a. Folliculitis (red arrow) and syncytium formation (black arrow) of the epithelial cells of a hair follicle. **b.** Sebaceous glands with syncytium formation (black arrow) in the epithelial cells (Favrot et al., 2005). (Favrot et al., 2005)

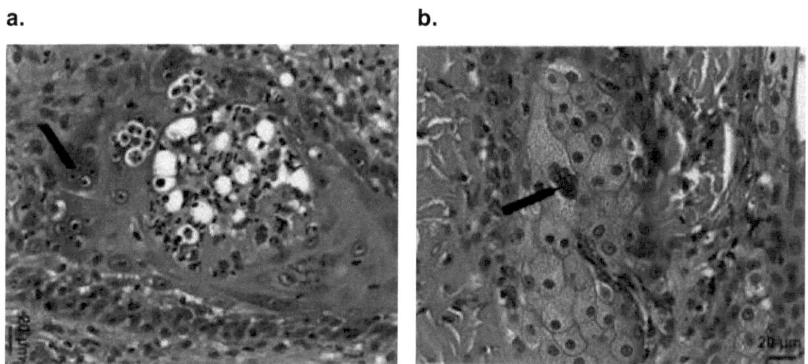

6.7.1.5.2. EYE

It has been mentioned that a common cause of uveitis is FeLV, the virus can cause lymphosarcoma and the uvea is considered to be the primary site of metastasis because transformed lymphocytes invade the eyeball through the uvea and cause uveitis (**Fig.14**), this will cause thickening and distortion of the iris, other signs may include iridocyclitis, hypopyon, hyphema, posterior synechiae, adhesions of the iris to the lens (**Fig. 15 and 16**), secondary glaucoma caused by infiltration and obstruction of the iridocorneal angle by tumour cells, chorioretinitis, spastic pupil syndrome (**Fig. 17**), retinal detachment and retinal detachment (**Fig. 17**), retinal detachment (**Fig. 18)** and retinal detachment (**Fig. 19). 17**), retinal detachment or chorioretinal masses; other ocular signs may include keratitis, orbital, eyelid, nictitating membrane and subconjunctival masses, and tumours in the anterior chamber and anterior uvea, e.g. iridal nodules (**Fig. 18**) and pinkish-white masses in the anterior chamber or attached to the anterior iris (Aroch et al., 2008; Colitz, 2005; Quiroz, 2019)..

Neurological signs with ophthalmic presentation such as anisocoria, mydriasis, central blindness or Horner's syndrome have also been described in FeLV-infected cats, most of these signs are caused by lymphoma and lymphocytic infiltrates in the brain or spinal cord, This neurotoxicity may be due to the fact that FeLV envelope glycoproteins can produce increased free intracellular calcium leading to neuronal death, which has also been described in HIV-infected humans. A FeLV envelope polypeptide was also found to cause neurotoxicity and FeLV-C was found to be significantly more neurotoxic than the same peptide derived from a FeLV-A subtype (Hartmann, 2012a). (Hartmann, 2012a).

Figure 14. a. Bilateral uveitis in cat with FeLV-positive generalised lymphadenomegaly. **b.** Right eyeball of the same cat showing abundant mucopurulent discharge, conjunctival hyperemia, diffuse corneal oedema, hyperemia with iris surface irregularities and persistent miosis (Quiroz, 2019). (Quiroz, 2019)

a.

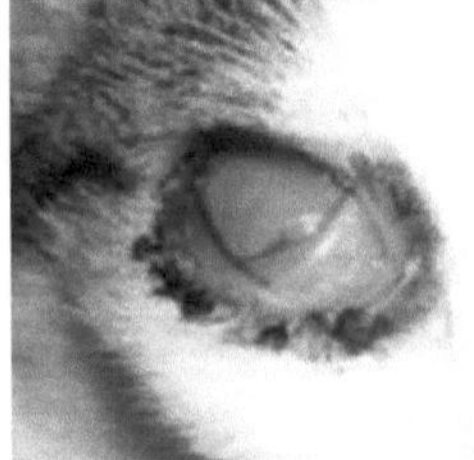

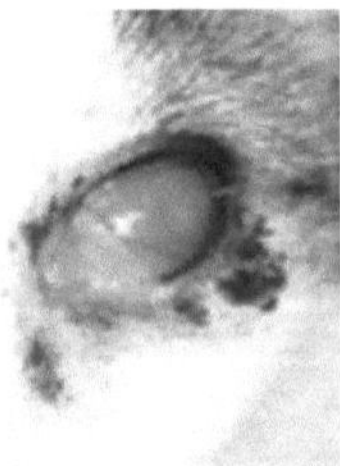

b.

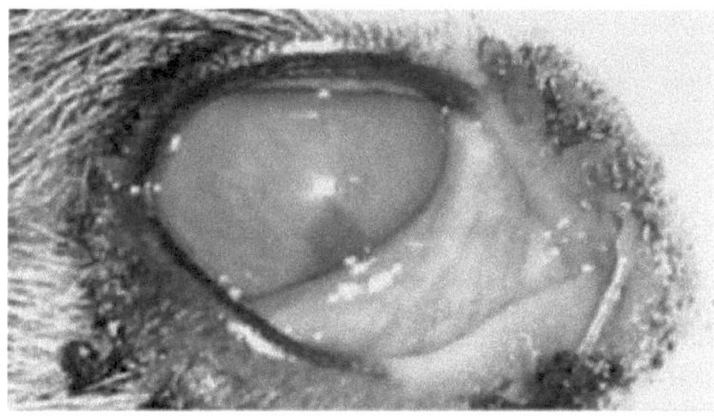

Figure 15. Right eyeball of a cat with uveitis. Hyperemia of the iris and pupil with dyskoria due to posterior synechiae is observed, hyphema is also observed. (Quiroz, 2019)

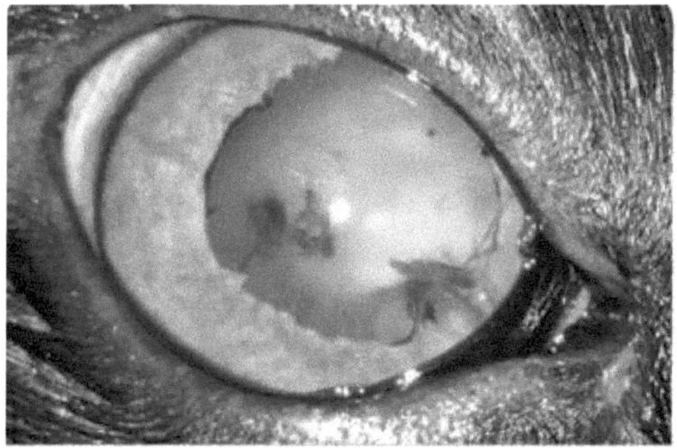

Figure 16. The right eye shows keratic precipitates while the left eye shows a hyphema blocking the tapetum lucidum reflex. (Quiroz, 2019).

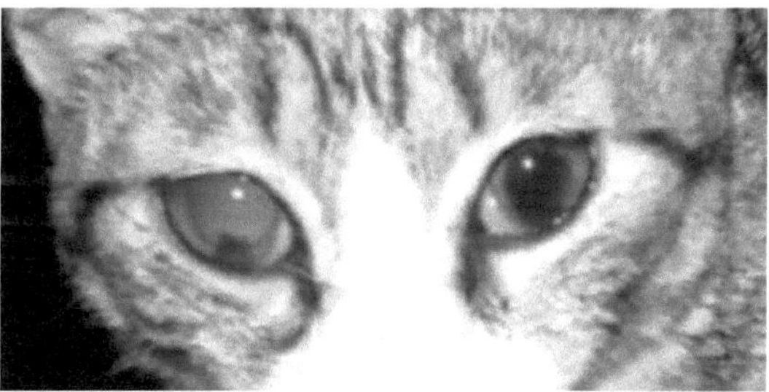

Figure 17. Spastic pupil syndrome. Anisocoria due to myiasis of the right eye that persisted in dark conditions. (Quiroz, 2019).

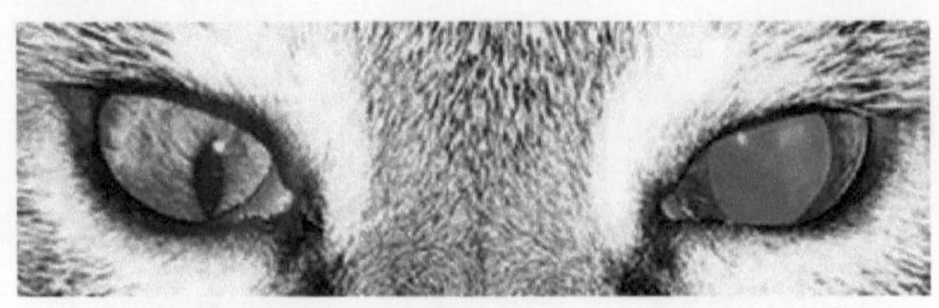

Figure 18. Multifocal grey masses on the iris surface of a 12-year-old FeLV-seropositive male cat. Histopathology confirmed the diagnosis of lymphoma (Aroch et al., 2008). (Aroch et al., 2008)..

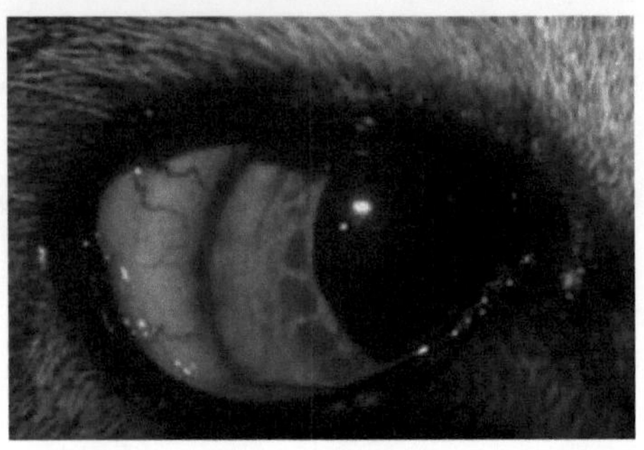

6.7.1.5.3. GENITOURINARY SYSTEM

FeLV has been recovered from urine and bladder epithelium; and FeLV-associated multicentric lymphoma of the kidneys and other kidney conditions have also been described (Hardy, 1981; Jarrett et al., 1973). (Hardy, 1981; Jarrett et al., 1973)..

Cats infected with FIV or FeLV are more likely to be diagnosed with immune-complex glomerulonephritis (ICGN), especially those with FeLV-induced haematopoietic neoplasms; this glomerular damage may be because FeLV continuously produces viral antigens, these plus host antibodies cause immune complex formation and deposition, the immune complexes consist of whole virus particles, gp70, p27, or p15E proteins, coupled to IgG (Glick et al., 1978; Hartmann, 2012a; Rossi et al., 2019; Tuomari et al., 1984)..

6.7.1.5.4. MAMMARY GLAND

As discussed in previous chapters, FeLV can be sequestered in some parts of the body, there are reports of females with focal mammary reactivation, these secrete the infectious virus in milk, so it is possible that puppies can be infected by this route, the first few days the viral antigen or infectious virus is not detected in blood, However, 45 days after FeLV neutralising antibodies passively acquired from colostrum decline, puppies may become viraemic, so puppies may develop infection 7 weeks after birth or 2 weeks after weaning. Although it is not yet known exactly how the virus enters through the mucosa, it is theorised that it may enter through lesions in the mucous membranes, it is also thought that the virus may interact with mucosal dendritic cells or intestinal M-cells, which are thought to mediate infection of T-lymphocytes with retroviruses; Finally, the virus may cross the gastrointestinal epithelium before physiological closure of the neonatal gut occurs; it is possible that these routes may be used by FeLV and HIV during the postnatal period (Hardy, 1993; Hardy, 1993). (Hardy, 1993; Hardy et al., 1976; Hartmann, 1998; Pacitti et al., 1986; Sellon et al., 1994)..

6.7.1.6. MOLECULAR FACTORS

6.7.1.6.1.1. INFLAMMATION

Bone marrow macrophages play an important role in regulating haematopoiesis by synthesising a number of stimulatory and inhibitory cytokines. Viral infections in macrophages can stimulate the release of a variety of cytokines, including prostaglandin E-2, interleukin-6 (IL-6) and tumour necrosis factor α (TNFα) (Khan et al., 1993)..

FeLV infection produces an altered cytokine network, feline retroviruses have been reported to alter cytokine (virokine) mRNA levels, these changes may result in specific alterations in cellular function and contribute to retroviral pathogenesis, these observations infer that altered cytokine expression patterns play a causal role in detrimental tissue inflammatory reactions and/or ineffective systemic immune responses; increased TNFα and decreased IL-2 and IL-4 have been described in some cats (Hartmann, 2014; Linen, 2014). (Hartmann, 2014; Linenberger & Deng, 1999)..

6.7.1.6.1.2. PROINFLAMMATORY CYTOKINES (IL-1,6, TUMOUR NECROSIS FACTOR α)

TNFα is a cytokine involved in the regulation of inflammation, immune reaction and erythropoiesis; it is synthesised mainly by activated macrophages, monocytes and other cells of the immune system. Although its exact function is not known, it is known to be the main mediator of septic shock and to be responsible for cachexia in chronic diseases by suppressing lipoprotein lipase in adipocytes *in vitro*, because it acts as the main mediator in the pathogenesis of infection, tissue injury and inflammation. (Goh, 1990; Odeh, 1990).. Increased TNFα production has been associated with retroviral infections, such as *human immunodeficiency virus* (HIV) and *simian immunodeficiency virus* (SIV) (Khan et al., 1993). (Khan et al., 1993)..

Macrophages are target cells for FeLV C, as this subtype has been found to be highly expressed in macrophages, in contrast to FeLV A. FeLV C-infected macrophages produce higher amounts of TNFα, especially in fibroblast and bone marrow macrophage cultures, although a high level of FeLV expression has also been described in macrophages infected with this subtype, which has been related to high levels of TNFα (Khan et al., 1993).. Similarly with HIV, TNFα has been shown to induce HIV expression *in vitro (*Folks et al., *1989)*. (Folks et al., 1989).

FeLV C-infected thymic lymphoma cells show increased proportions of palmitic acid, which has been shown to potentiate the effects of TNF α . (Bjerve et al., 1987).. Erythroid cells infected by FeLV C may acquire increased susceptibility to the inhibitory effects of TNFα through increased palmitate production and thus, by suppressing erythroid progenitors in the bone marrow of cats, FeLV C could induce erythroid aplasia (Khan et al., 1993).

Macrophage dysfunctions, including defects in monocyte-to-macrophage maturation have been reported in HIV patients, where increased TNFα has been linked to anaemia and lymphopenia, as well as inhibiting human B cell differentiation, and TNFα has also been found to be elevated in serum in 50% of patients who developed AIDS (Kashiwa et al., 1987; Lähdevirta et al., 1988;

Maury & Lăhdevirta, 1990). (Kashiwa et al., 1987; Lähdevirta et al., 1988; Maury & Lăhdevirta, 1990).. Based on these and other observations, it was proposed that treatment of AIDS patients should include TNFα antagonists (Lehmann et al. antagonists (Lehmann et al., 1992).

IL-1 has been suggested to be involved in the regulation of the production of human erythroid progenitors (Zucali et al., 1987). IL-1 also potentiates the lethal effects of TNFα. TNFα and IL-1 can be released in a co-ordinated manner by activated macrophages and one can induce the production of the other. The inhibitory effect of IL-1 on feline erythroid progenitors has been evaluated and compared to TNFα, it has a mild effect on feline erythroid progenitors and a moderate effect on fibroblast progenitors. (Khan, 1992)..

6.7.1.6.1.3. SUPPLEMENT

Incubation of normal feline serum with FeLV has been reported to result in complement activation via the classical pathway, which could be the result of complement interaction with circulating immune complexes, demonstrated by consumption of C1, C4, C2, C3 and, to a lesser extent, C3 components, however these observations also indicated inefficient virolysis of FeLV by normal cat serum, However, these observations also indicated inefficient virolysis of FeLV by normal cat serum, so it is thought that there may be a factor present that contributes to the relative ease with which horizontal FeLV infection in cats occurs (Kobilinsky et al. (Kobilinsky et al., 1980)..

Primate sera, including humans, lyse retroviruses in the apparent absence of antibodies as a result of complement activation. It has therefore been suggested that in higher mammals complement provides a natural defence mechanism that inhibits or interferes with retrovirus infection and replication. Furthermore, the relative efficacy of complement-mediated virolysis has been shown to correlate with primate phylogeny (Sherwin et al., 1978; Welsh et al., 1976).. In contrast, sera from lower mammals such as rodents are unable to lyse retroviruses. The ineffectiveness of feline sera in lysing FeLV indicates that this species also falls into this latter category (Kobilinsky et al., 1980)..

6.7.1.6.1.4. INTERFERON

Interferons (INF) are cytokines with different biological functions and are classified into type I, II and III IFNs. IFN-I are produced by virus-infected cells and are known as "viral INF", their induction is regulated by the classical and Toll-like receptor (TLR) pathway, they have non-specific antiviral activity and participate in the innate defence mechanism, They also induce enzymes that degrade viral messenger RNA and thus inhibit viral replication in neighbouring cells or the cell that produces them, they also induce apoptosis of cells with genetic damage or uncontrolled proliferation and of virus-infected cells, which limits the spread from one cell to another; INF-I has been shown to inhibit the release of retroviral particles by interfering with the processing of viral proteins and their assembly into complete virions, resulting in defective, non-infectious virus particles. INF can also be an effective bridge between innate and adaptive immunity, as it can promote the differentiation and function of various types of immune cells such as dendritic cells (DC), NK, B cells, CD4+ and CD8+ T cells; furthermore, INF-I can induce anti-proliferative and anti-inflammatory responses, as well as increase the expression of MHC class I molecules in all cells, which contributes to the elimination of infected cells. (Akira & Uematsu, 2007; Ballesteros et al., 2011; Cattori et al., 2011; Collado et al., 2007; Collado et al., 2009; Montaraz C, 2012)..

There are different types of INF-I, these are IFN-α, IFN-β, and IFN-ω, among others, and their cellular source varies, IFN-β is produced by various non-hematopoietic cells, IFN-α and IFN-ω are produced by haematopoietic cells. The latter is secreted by virus-infected leukocytes and has antiviral, antiproliferative and immunomodulatory effects, is involved in the non-specific response based on increased expression of several acute phase proteins and MHC-I molecules; up-regulates phagocytic activity of red blood cells, macrophages, NK cells and decreases recurrent viral excretion (Chang et al., 2018; Krause et al., 2004; Sen, 2001).

INF is currently used as an immunotherapeutic for retroviral infections in human and feline medicine. Human IFN-α (HuINF-α) was first used in cats for its antiviral and immune modulating properties, however, IFN's are species specific and neutralising antibodies develop several weeks after initiation of therapy and require high doses of INF to develop, making this therapy ineffective in the long term. These problems can be overcome with the administration of a feline-specific INF (FeINF) (Ballesteros et al., 2011; Leal & Gil, 2016)..

Several subtypes of recombinant FeINF-α (rFeINF-α) have been described that could have similar benefits to those seen in humans, such as in the treatment of chronic viral diseases and various tumours in cats, however, it is not yet available for clinical use. The only commercially available recombinant FeINF-ω (rFeINF-ω) is frequently used to treat viral infections. Cats with FeLV treated with it have shown significant clinical improvement and increased lifespan, but proviral load and viraemia did not change, suggesting that rFeINF-ω has no antiviral effect, but may have a possible modulation of the innate system; rFeINF-ω is known to affect the downregulation of retrotranscriptase (RT) activity, affecting the FeLV cycle, decrease the viability of infected cells and suppress the processing or assembly of viral proteins and/or the release of virions in the late stages of maturation (Ballesteros et al., 2011; Collado et al., 2007; Wonderling et al., 2002)..

6.7.1.6.1.5. TOLL-LIKE RECEPTORS (TLR)

The immune system needs to regulate its activation as inappropriate or unregulated activation can be detrimental to health, so pathogen detection is mediated by several families of proteins called pattern recognition receptors (PRRs) and these bind to pathogen-associated molecular patterns (PAMPs). Toll-like receptors (TLRs) are part of the PRRs. TLR3 recognises viral components on the cell surface and TLR3, TLR7, TLR8, TLR9 recognise viral components because they are located in endosomal compartments and detect nucleic acids, so a virus must be internalised and transported to the endosomal compartment where they are degraded by host cell enzymes, releasing the viral nucleic acid. Once it is recognised, intrinsic signalling pathways are activated and induce IFN-I (Akira & Uematsu, 2007; Browne, 2020)..

Although TLRs generally induce a protective immune response, there are cases in which they can be used by viruses and contribute to pathogenesis, as in the case of HIV-1 where TLRs contribute to recognition and elimination, but can also induce cytokine secretion that favours a chronic proinflammatory state, viral replication and dissemination of virions. Another case is that of TLR3, which is thought to play a role in tumour formation induced by Moloney murine leukaemia and FeLV, as it can activate NFκB signalling via the U3 region of TLR; it has anti-apoptosis and growth-promoting activity and has therefore been implicated in leukaemogenesis, suggesting a role for TLR3 in tumour formation (Beyaert et al. (Beyaert et al., 2008; Hernandez et al., 2007)..

6.7.1.6.1.6. MAJOR HISTOCOMPATIBILITY COMPLEX (MHC)

These molecular markers give the individual a tissue identity that is recognised by the immune system and encode class I and II antigens that participate in the induction of the immunospecific response by presenting the antigen to T lymphocytes. MHC molecules arrive at the cell membrane bound to self elements, so when presented to T cells they do not activate them, however, if there are pathological or infectious changes in the cell and they carry a foreign molecule instead of a self molecule, the T cell is activated and responds immediately. Class I (MHC-I) presents antigens of viral or tumour origin to Tc-CD8+ (cytotoxic) cells; and Class II (MHC-II) presents intravesicular or exogenous antigens to Th-CD4+ (helper) cells. (Mach et al., 1996; Vega Robledo, 2009; Yuhki et al., 2008).

The distribution of MHC-II in the domestic cat has been characterised in various tissues and in peripheral blood mononuclear cells, and is expressed not only by antigen-presenting cells but also by T lymphocytes. In cats persistently infected with FeLV, abnormalities in MHC-II expression by T lymphocytes were observed, suggesting that chronic virus stimulation could be responsible for sustained elevations in MHC-II expression (Rideout et al., 1992)..

6.7.1.7. CELLULAR FACTORS

6.7.1.7.1.1. EOSINOPHILES

They are dual function cells serving as modulators of inflammation and as phagocytic, cytotoxic and antigen processing cells, however, their involvement in FeLV infection is not yet defined, but in retrovirus infections such as HIV it is known that eosinophils may act as a cellular reservoir of virus that may be difficult to reach with antiviral drugs. (Wooley et al., 2000)..

Eosinophilic leukaemia is rare in cats and there are only two reports of FeLV involvement in this type of leukaemia, the first report was of a cat that was experimentally infected with an *env* gene recombinant feline retrovirus (PR8) and it is suspected that changes in the virus envelope may have altered its pathogenicity and caused this type of leukaemia; The second case was an ELISA positive FeLV-positive cat, the haemogram showed leukocytosis with 77% eosinophils and cytological examination of bone marrow, liver, lymph node and spleen aspirates revealed a predominance of mature and immature eosinophils. References in the literature indicate that most cats with eosinophilic leukaemia are negative for FeLV, but this does not rule out the possibility that the virus may remain latent in bone marrow and induce a genetic alteration in haematopoietic stem cells (Gelain et al., 2006; Lewis et al., 1985; Sharifi et al., 2007)..

6.7.1.7.1.2. NEUTROPHILES

They phagocytose and degrade the invading organism using the contents of the lysosome through two mechanisms, oxygen-independent and oxygen-dependent. FeLV affects neutrophil function, believed to be due to the insertion of proviral sequences, which would result in a progeny of physiologically and structurally altered cells, these changes affect the chemotactic and phagocytic capacity of neutrophils, some alterations are reduction in the production of reactive oxygen species (ROS), interference in protein interactions or cause fundamental changes in protein structure (Lafrado & Olsen, 1986; Wardini et al., 2010)..

Protein kinase C (PKC) is a cytoplasmic enzyme that regulates many processes in the neutrophil, including the respiratory burst, one of the substrates of PKC is the enzyme NADPH oxidase, when Ca ions are mobilised^{2+} , the NADPH/NADH oxidase system is activated, which reduces molecular oxygen to form superoxide anions (O_2), which are used by the neutrophil for microbicidal activity. How FeLV interferes with neutrophil activity has not yet been elucidated, whether it directly decreases PKC or NADPH oxidase activation is not known, but FeLV-p15E is thought to possibly suppress cell functions by altering Ca^{2+} mobilisation (Dezzutti et al., 1989)..

6.7.1.7.1.3. MACROPHAGES

They are located in all major compartments of the body and monitor effectively, suggesting that viral particles tend to be taken up by macrophages in the early stages of infection and once digested can delay or even prevent the spread of infection to susceptible cells, however, the virus can replicate in macrophages and spread to organs and tissues, and infected monocytes in the circulation can spread the infection by their migration through the body, thus macrophages may play a crucial role for the outcome of the infection (Mims, 1964; Mogens, 1964). (Mims, 1964; Mogensen, 1979)..

Impaired macrophage function is known to increase the susceptibility of cats to FeLV, with experimental administration of corticosteroids it has been noted that macrophage activity decreases, resulting in failure to contain the infection in the early stages, viral replication in lymphoid tissues and development of disease, so it is thought that macrophages may act as effector cells against FeLV, as initiators of the immune response through antigen presentation and other cooperative mechanisms of lymphocytes (Hoover et al., 1981; Ogilvie et al., 1988; Ogilvie et al., 1988). (Hoover et al., 1981; Ogilvie et al., 1988)..

Macrophages from young cats are more susceptible and have a higher rate of replication in lymphocytes than adult cats, and it is believed that this is because in adults macrophages mature to an effective response against retrovirus (Hoover et al., 1981; Rojko et al., 1979)..

6.7.1.7.1.4. CYTOTOXIC CELLS

NK cells are lymphocytes of the innate immune system and kill cancer and virus-infected cells by expressing multiple receptors on the cell surface that allow them to recognise infected or transformed cells, and upon identification and activation of the target cell NK cells produce cytokines (such as INF-α) releasing cytotoxic granules containing granzymes and perforins to induce apoptosis of target cells. NK activation during viral infections depends on cytokines and interaction with other immune cells, and their immediate activation is very important for the control of these infections. However, it is known that the Friend retrovirus (FV) in mice can manipulate molecular or cellular factors that suppress the NK cell response, so that NK cells lack cytokines for effective activation, and the virus is known to inhibit the expression of the ligand by which NK cells recognise infected cells; In another experiment, a synthetic peptide (CKS-17) with homology to a region of p15E conserved among numerous retroviruses was used, which was observed to almost completely decrease the ability of NK cells to respond to IFN-α, so it is thought that this may be a mechanism of immunosuppression by inhibiting their function; Despite this information on the interaction of retroviruses with NK cells, the role of these cells in FeLV infection is not clear, as there is no recent information and the last published study was that of Kooistra & Splitter in 1985 where they mention that NK cells do not have an important role in the immune defence against FeLV, however we could think that their interaction is similar to that of the retroviruses already mentioned (Guven et al. (Guven et al., 2005; Harris et al., 1987; Kooistra & Splitter, 1985; Littwitz-Salomon et al., 2016; Littwitz-Salomon et al., 2018; Vieira et al., 2022)..

6.7.2. ORGANS AND CELLS OF THE IMMUNE RESPONSE

The target cell of FeLV is the monocyte-macrophage and many researchers have reported abnormalities in the adaptive immune response, such as reduced paracortical lymphocytes in lymphonodes, thymic atrophy, leukopenia and leukocyte dysfunction. An example of this is FeLV-induced immunodeficiency syndrome, or FeLV-FAIDS, the gp-70 gene induces immunodeficiency, and influences $CD4^{+}$ and T-lymphocyte-dependent antibody responsiveness, leading to the development of fatal immune deficiency syndrome. (Ackley et al., 1990; Ogilvie et al., 1988)..

Atrophy of lymphoid tissues is often accompanied by lymphopenia, and secondary disorders occurring in these cats may include anaemia, enteritis (myeloblastopenia), general debilitation, feline infectious peritonitis, chronic non-healing wounds and skin abscesses, chronic gingivitis and stomatitis, and chronic upper respiratory disease. (Hardy, 1982)..

6.7.2.1. PRIMARY: THYMUS, BONE MARROW

6.7.2.1.1. TIMO

Kittens infected prenatally or neonatally with FeLV have a higher mortality rate and develop marked thymic atrophy, termed "fainting kitten syndrome", leading to severe immunosuppression and early death. (Hartmann, 2012a). Many infected kittens develop a dwarfism syndrome with growth retardation, thymic atrophy and death between 8 and 12 weeks of age. FeLV replicates best in rapidly dividing cells, so it replicates in large numbers in thymic lymphocytes and destroys them, resulting in an impaired immune response leading to predisposition to secondary infectious diseases. These kittens often develop septicaemia, upper respiratory tract disease, pneumonia and generalised skin infections that can lead to death. It is not known whether thymic atrophy is mediated by an autoaggressive mechanism, such as that occurring in MuLV-infected mice, or by direct lymphocytolysis (Hardy, 1982)..

6.7.2.1.2. BONE MARROW

As discussed above, the bone marrow can be altered by FeLV, leading to myelosuppression or myelodysplasia, haematological changes such as regenerative or non-regenerative anaemia, persistent, transient or cyclic neutropenia due to myeloid hypoplasia at all granulocytic stages leading to alterations in neutrophil precursors; thrombocytopenia and platelet function abnormalities, aplastic anaemia (pancytopenia), panleukopenia-like syndrome and maturation arrest in myelocyte and metamyelocyte stages. These alterations are caused because the cells of the bone marrow microenvironment provide a reservoir for FeLV where the provirus can be latent in myelomonocytic progenitor cells and stromal fibroblasts, the provirus can inactivate genes in these cells, alter the expression of neighbouring genes or induce the expression of antigens on the cell surface leading to their immune-mediated destruction. In addition to these changes, it is known that exposure of the bone marrow to some strains of the virus can cause suppression of erythrogenesis and chronic inflammation due to high cytokine concentration (Abdollahi-Pirbahi-Pirbahi). (Abdollahi-Pirbazari et al., 2019; Hartmann, 2012a; Stützer et al., 2010)..

6.7.2.2. LYMPHOID ORGANS

6.7.2.2.1. LYMPHONODOS

Lymphatic atrophy and hyperplasia are present in FeLV-infected cats. Lymph nodes may be small with a marked reduction in lymphocytes in the paracortical area, these areas may be occupied with reticular cells and some lymphocytes, and as a result of atrophy of lymphoid tissues there may be lymphopenia. Lymphoid depletion also occurs in Peyer's patches and many infected cats develop chronic enteritis. However, in cats with secondary infections there is follicular hyperplasia, congestion and infiltration of plasma cells, neutrophils and histiocytes in the medullary zone of the lymph nodes (Hardy, 1982)..

6.7.2.2.2. BAZO

Lymphoid changes of the spleen are less marked than lymph node changes in FeLV-infected cats. Follicular hyperplasia is occasionally seen with secondary infections. Some cats show reduction of the entire white pulp (Hardy, 1982).

6.7.3.CELL-MEDIATED IMMUNITY

Cytotoxic T-lymphocytes (CTL) are among the first defence mechanisms in response to viral and retroviral infections, play a role in elimination and replication control in persistent infections and may determine the outcome of infection. FeLV can have a silencing effect on humoral immunity, resulting in undetectable or very low levels of neutralising antibodies in persistently viraemic cats. A similar effect occurs in the cellular response, as cytotoxic T-lymphocyte activity is observed up to 4 to 7 weeks after exposure to the virus, CD4+ and CD8+ T-lymphocytes are lost and infected T-lymphocytes produce low levels of lymphocyte-stimulating factors. This temporary delay and disruption in immune mechanisms may allow the virus to infect a greater number of cells. It has also been observed that recognition of cytotoxic T cells for *gag/pro* (protease, PT) occurs 4 to 7 weeks after exposure and for *env* it occurs 10 to 13 weeks after exposure. This recognition time is independent of infection outcome (Flynn et al., 2002; Hartmann, 2012a)..

Although the exact immunosuppressive properties of FeLV are not yet understood, the p15E envelope peptide is believed to inhibit T and B cell function, alter morphology, interfere with lymphocyte cytotoxic response, IL-2 and macrophage activating factor (MAF) production and accumulation (Copelan et al., 1983; Mathes et al., 1979; Orosz et al., 1985; Orosz et al., 1985). (Copelan et al., 1983; Mathes et al., 1979; Orosz et al., 1985)..

6.7.3.1. HUMORAL IMMUNITY

Induction of neutralising antibodies can prevent infection prior to provirus integration into the cell and persistence, they neutralise only one serotype (FeLV A, B or C), i.e. A will not neutralise B. Their main targets are the SU surface proteins gp70, envelope and transmembrane TM p15E of which immunosuppressive properties are described, antibodies to gp73, p58 and p27 have also been reported (Denner et al., 2010; Harder, 1982; Harder, 1982). (Denner et al., 2010; Hardy, 1982).. Binding of the antibodies to gp70 blocks the attachment of the virus to cell receptors or disrupts the penetration process, thus preventing infection (Ginel Perez et al., 2010; Hardy, 1982). (Ginel Perez et al., 1996).. The integration of the p15E antigen into vaccines has been proposed as immunosuppressive activity correlates with viral load, so it is thought unlikely that the small amount of p15E in the vaccine would cause immunosuppression, however, although antibody production against this protein was observed in immunised cats, some others infected with FeLV and having high titres of antibodies to the p15E protein, little involvement in virus neutralisation was observed, so it may not present any benefit in immunisation (Langhammer et al., 1996). (Langhammer et al., 2005; Langhammer et al., 2006)..

Antibody levels are related to the speed of recovery from infection, as cats that develop high levels of FeLV antibodies have no or brief viraemia, as opposed to cats with low levels that have persistent infection, however, there are cats with a prolonged viraemic phase that recovered from infection after developing low or moderate levels of antibodies. Cats that terminated infection approximately 2 weeks after developing viraemia had high levels of antibodies to all viral components and many of these were to the gp73, p58, p27, p24, and p15E antigens, unlike those that did not have a prolonged viral phase. This proves that the amount of antibodies against specific virus components is as important as the total amount of antibodies against all components, and it is theorised that there are two mechanisms that aid in the termination of infection, the primary mechanism being based on the neutralising capacity of the virus and the second on the activity of antibodies against infected cells Higgins, 1980.

Another type of antibody that may appear after exposure to the virus is antibody to FOCMA, an acronym for *Feline Oncornavirus-associated Cell Membrane Antigen*, which is present in the membrane of neoplastic cells. Cats with antibody to FOCMA are at low risk of developing neoplasia (Ginel Perez et al., 1996; Jarret & Russell, 1978)..

Neutralising antibodies and cytotoxic T lymphocytes are important in protecting cats against FeLV, but in most cases neutralising antibodies were present once cats with transient viraemia recovered, unlike specific cytotoxic T lymphocytes which were present one week after exposure, and cats immunised with a DNA vaccine were protected from infection without developing virus neutralising antibodies; so antibodies stop the spread of virus and establish resistance to infection, cell-mediated immunity is likely to take over the elimination of already infected cells and protect against the development of latent infection (Cattori et al., 2007a). (Argyl et al., 2001).

6.7.4.DIAGNOSTIC TESTS

Tests that can be performed quickly in the clinic are point of care ELISA (POC) or rapid immunomigration test (RIM) are the first to be performed and use serum, plasma or whole blood, tears and saliva should not be used, they detect soluble p27 antigen at day 30 after FeLV exposure and have shown good sensitivity and specificity. Maternal and vaccinal immunity do not interfere with the test. If the result is positive or thought to be a false positive it should be confirmed with follow-up tests such as FeLV p27 antigen microplate ELISA, polymerase chain reaction (PCR) test or immunofluorescent antibody (IFA) test, although a POC test from a different manufacturer can also be used (Little et al. (Little et al., 2020; St Denis, 2022)..

IFA detects p27 antigen and other structural core antigens in the cytoplasm of cells, detects secondary viraemia when the bone marrow is infected and if there is insufficient antigen production the infection is not detected; in clinical practice peripheral blood is used, but cytology of bone marrow and other tissues can also be used (Little et al., 2020; St Denis, 2022)..

PCR amplifies and detects viral genetic material, proviral DNA or viral RNA by pairing short genetic fragments and detects very small amounts of viral genetic material. Diagnostic laboratories increasingly offer PCR assays on whole blood, bone marrow and other tissues, and help to resolve conflicting test results if a positive result is obtained (**Table 3**). (Little et al., 2020; St Denis, 2022)..

Table 3. Variations in CRP. Modified from (Little et al., 2020; St Denis, 2022; Stone et al., 2020).

Type of PCR	Specifications
Real-time PCR	Sensitive and fast, it can use whole blood, bone marrow and other tissues to help detect regressed cats.
Quantitative real-time PCR	It helps to classify the course of infection, < 1 million copies/ml proviral DNA is more likely to be a regressive patient, and with ≥1 million copies/ml proviral DNA is likely to be a progressive patient.
Real-time DNA PCR	It is highly sensitive and specific, detects provirus in peripheral blood, can detect progressive and regressive cats.
Proviral PCR	Detects provirus in the peripheral blood or bone marrow of cats 1-2 weeks after exposure to the virus, detects regressively infected cats.
Reverse Transcriptase PCR (RT-PCR)	It detects viral RNA in saliva and is a reliable parameter of antigenemia, helping to classify the course of infection, this test can detect infection 1-3 weeks after exposure.
Real-time RT-PCR	Detects viral RNA one week after FeLV exposure.

As mentioned in the topic on Course of infection, it is important to be aware of the different courses of FeLV presentation in order to correctly interpret the results of diagnostic tests and apply them appropriately to determine infection in cats (**Figure 19**).

Progressive infection is usually confirmed by repeated POC tests that detect the p27 antigen indicating antigenemia, so repeat testing several weeks or months apart, usually 16 weeks, is necessary as positive results indicate progressive infection. However, during early infection when host-virus balance is not yet present, some cats may alternate between positive and negative results (referred to as "alternating"). (Hofmann-Lehmann & Hartmann, 2020; Little et al., 2020).. This infection is accompanied by persistence of proviral DNA which is detected by PCR, and if proviral load is measured by quantitative PCR, a high viral load is observed (Hofmann-Lehmann & Hartmann, 2020; Little et al., 2020). (Hartmann, 2012a).

Cats with regressed infection will test negative no later than 16 weeks post infection, PCR can detect provirus in blood from antigen-negative regressed infected cats; they are also associated with a low proviral DNA load, and although these cats are likely to never clear the infection, proviral loads may fall below the limit of detection, this also depends on the sensitivity of the PCR, however other tests where cats are RNA viral positive have been shown to be more susceptible to reactivate the virus than RNA viral negative cats (Hofmann-Lehmann & Hartmann, 2020; Little et al, 2020). (Hofmann-Lehmann & Hartmann, 2020; Little et al., 2020)..

During abortive infection, the cat manages to stop infection before provirus integration and all tests for antigen, viral RNA and proviral DNA are negative, making the presence of antibodies the only indication of infection. (Hofmann-Lehmann & Hartmann, 2020; Little et al., 2020)..

In focal infection, p27 antigen may be present in the blood, but the isolation of infectious virus is negative, if this persists for years this is because the cat's immune system keeps virus replication isolated in certain tissues, so that antigen may be produced intermittently or minimally, resulting in weakly positive or discordant antigen tests, which may alternate between positive and negative results. (Hartmann, 2012a; Hofmann-Lehmann & Hartmann, 2020)..

Figure 19. The European Advisory Board on Cat Diseases (ABCD) diagnostic tool for FeLV. Modified from (Hofmann-Lehmann & Hartmann, 2020)

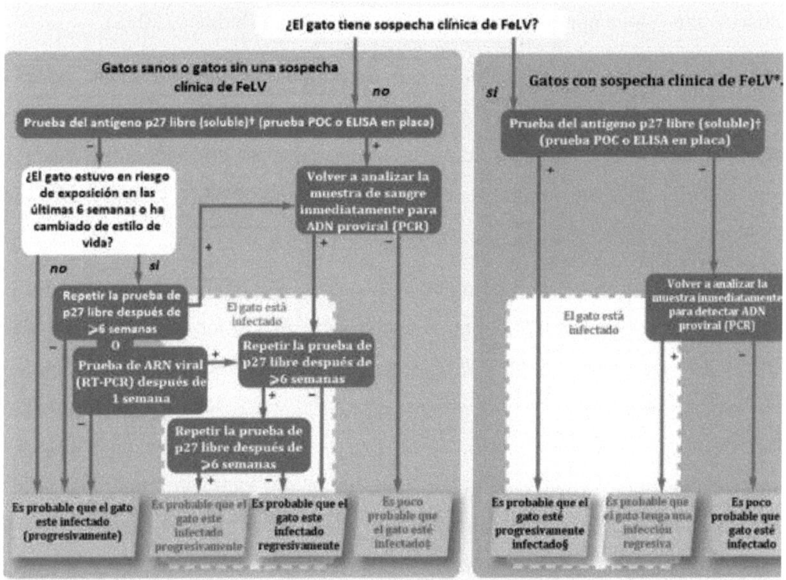

†Whenever analysis of free FeLV p27 antigen in blood samples (POC or plaque ELISA) is suggested in any of the steps of the algorithm, analysis of viral RNA in saliva samples (RT-PCR) may alternatively be used. ‡**In** very rare cases, focal FeLV infection may result in a positive free p27 antigen and negative provirus PCR result in blood samples. §**In** cats with a clinical suspicion of FeLV infection and a positive free p27 antigen test, a confirmatory test is not required as a false positive test is less likely in these cats; the positive predictive value is high as the cats are already in the group with a high risk of FeLV infection.

6.7.5. FELV-ASSOCIATED VIRAL ONCOGENESIS

Proto-oncogenes are genes encoding growth-promoting proteins and **oncogenes** are their mutated versions that allow cells to become "self-sufficient". Insertional mutagenesis is the cause of FeLV-induced neoplasms; the virus has a promoter gene that inserts near a proto-oncogene (commonly *myc*), altering it and transforming it into an oncogene, leading to uncontrolled proliferation. Table 4 shows the loci where FeLV is commonly integrated and the neoplasms where they are frequently identified (Fujino et al., 2008; Modiano, 2013)..

FeLV subgroups influence the biodiversity of strains, as subgroup A and B can combine with *myc* or TCR to create FeLV-MYC or FeLV-TCR, which are considered tumour-producing. The Rickard strain of FeLV (FeLV-R) integrates close to the *c-myc* gene causing its overexpression. (Modiano, 2013)..

The RNA sequences of exFeLV can introduce the oncogene and form a recombinant virus such as FeLV-B or FeSV, which contain cells with oncogenic sequences, so recombinant viruses entering a new cell are oncogenic, which is why exFeLV has an important role in cat tumorigenesis. (Hartmann, 2012a; Modiano, 2013)..

The FeLV-A genome can recombine with cellular oncogenes resulting in FeSV containing one of several oncogenes such as *fes, fms or fgr*, during this process, part of the *gag* gene, *env* and all polar genes are lost, making FeSV dependent on FeLV for replication, so cats with FeSV are FeLV positive. Because there can be different recombinations with various proto-oncogenes, the result is a unique and distinct recombination in each isolate, yet all produce fibrosarcomas. These fibrosarcomas tend to grow rapidly and often have multiple locally invasive cutaneous or subcutaneous nodules and may metastasise to the lung and other sites. There are other fibrosarcomas with different characteristics to those caused by FeSV, and are classified as feline injection site sarcomas (FISS) which are caused by granulomatous inflammation following inoculation with adjuvanted vaccines, but neither FeSV nor FeLV is known to influence the development of FISS (Hartmann, 2012a; Modiano, 2013)..

Table 4. Common integration sites identified in FeLV-associated neoplasms (Fujino et al., 2008).

Locus	Tumour type
c-myc	T-cell lymphoid tumour (mainly thymic lymphoma)
flvi-1	Lymphoid tumour (splenic lymphoma)
flvi-2	T-cell lymphoid tumour (mainly thymic lymphoma)
fit-1	T-cell lymphoid tumour (mainly thymic lymphoma)
pim-1	T-cell lymphoid tumour (mainly thymic lymphoma)
flit-1	T-cell lymphoid tumour (thymic lymphoma)

6.7.6. VACCINATIONS AND VACCINATION

FeLV control necessarily requires a combination of actions such as identification of infected cats through diagnostic testing to separate them from susceptible cats, disinfection of positive cat sites, personalised vaccination schedules and frequent serological monitoring of serum antibody titres. (Sanchez Pacheco, 2019).

6.7.6.1. FACTORS TO CONSIDER IN ESTABLISHING A VACCINATION SCHEDULE

Vaccine-induced adaptive immunity is influenced by an interaction of factors unique to each patient, it is impossible to predict the outcome of vaccination or exposure to a pathogen and vaccination should never be offered as a guarantee of protection. The risk of infection and the development of disease depends on a number of factors, including age, health status, extent of exposure to the virus, geographical prevalence of infection and vaccination history; factors that adversely affect the ability to respond to vaccination include maternally derived antibody (MDA) interference, congenital or acquired immunodeficiency, concurrent disease or infection, inadequate nutrition, immunosuppressive drugs, chronic stress and immunosenescence, an ageing immune response in geriatric individuals. Age is an important element in assessing an individual's risk profile, as infectious diseases are more prevalent in kittens and those under 6 months of age than in adult cats, so kittens represent a prime target population for vaccination. MDA provide important protection to the kitten, but can also interfere with or neutralise vaccines, as MDA levels vary in individuals, the age at which the kitten will respond to vaccination will also vary, and it is believed that the most common cause of vaccination failure in kittens is vaccination too early (when MDA is still interfering). Another cause to consider in setting the vaccination schedule is population density and exposure to other cats (nurseries, catteries, foster or shelter), as these are factors that increase the risk of FeLV exposure; it should also be noted that the introduction of new individuals to the household is a potential risk to both the introduced cat and the group due to possible introduction of the virus and immunosuppression from stress generated by social change; and although indoor cats may be at low risk of contact with the virus they may be at risk due to fomites brought in by the owner (Ford et al., 2013). (Ford et al., 2013).

Table 5. Risk assessment variables that determine an individualised vaccination schedule. Modified from (Stone et al., 2020)

Risk factors	Considerations
Age and stage of life	Susceptibility, MDA, activity level, reproductive status
Health status	Coexisting diseases
FeLV exposure	Geographical prevalence, lifestyle, accommodation
History	Adverse events to vaccination, littermate response to vaccination, previous diseases
Immunodeficiency	Congenital or acquired (including chronic stress)

6.7.6.2. VACCINES AVAILABLE IN MEXICO

The aim of vaccination is to evoke an immune response that allows cats to recover from exposure to FeLV. A number of vaccines have been introduced to the market, which have been shown to offer protection against persistent viraemia, the use of these along with increased routine testing is likely responsible for the reduction in the prevalence of FeLV infection in the domestic cat population (Grosenbaugh et al., 2017).. Four vaccines are currently marketed in Mexico, two inactivated virus vaccines, Leukocell® 2 and Nobivac® Feline 2-FeLV, and two recombinant virus vaccines, PureVax Feline 4 FeLV® and Leucogen® (**Table 6**).

Leukocell® 2 is prepared from an FeLV-transformed lymphoid cell line that releases soluble viral particles in cell culture medium, induces antibodies against gp70, FOCMA and neutralising antibodies. (Zoetis, 2023). Anti-FOCMA is associated with protection against neoplastic disease, but its role in protection against persistent viraemia is unclear, however, this vaccine has been shown to protect against persistent viraemia for at least 12 months (Harbour et al., 2002). (Harbour et al., 2002).

Nobivac ® Feline 2-FeLV contains tissue culture-derived Feline Leukaemia virus subgroups A and B, the viral antigens have been chemically inactivated, studies indicate that this vaccine protects for two years against persistent viraemia; and although post-vaccination cats do not develop neutralising antibodies, it appears to prime them for a neutralising antibody response once they come into contact with FeLV, lower amounts of proviral DNA and plasma loads of viral RNA have also been observed (MSD, 2023; Patel et al., 2015; Pedersen, 1993). (MSD, 2023; Patel et al., 2015; Pedersen, 1993)..

PureVax Feline 4 FeLV® contains FeLV-A *env* and *gag* genes that have been inserted into the canaripox virus vector using recombinant DNA technology, and have been shown to provide protection against oronasal exposure, the use of live viral vectors is an alternative and the Canarypox Virus Vector (ALVAC) is one of the most studied, a natural property of ALVAC is that it can only multiply in avian species, making it safe for the vaccinated host and although it does not multiply in mammals and produce proteins from the FeLV genes (Paoletti, 1996; Patel et al., 2015; Poulet et al., 2003)..

Leucogen® which is another recombinant vaccine, but this is a subunit vaccine, i.e. this is the p45 protein moiety of *env*, the SU glycoprotein of the gp70 *env* envelope (Jarrett & Ganière, 1996; Langhammer et al., 2011). (Jarrett & Ganière, 1996; Langhammer et al., 2011)

Both recombinant vaccines induce neutralising antibodies, because they contain the envelope glycoprotein, which is probably involved in the elimination of free virus particles, and it has also been shown that the *env* and *gag* genes are targeted by cytotoxic T lymphocytes and are responsible for eliminating FeLV-infected cells. (Flynn et al., 2000; Poulet et al., 2003)..

Table 6. Vaccines currently available in Mexico for FeLV. Modified from (Aguilar B et al., 2019)..

Vaccine	Type of vaccine	Name	Content
Feline herpesvirus (HVF-1) Feline calicivirus (FVC) Feline viral panleukopenia (FVP) *C. felis* Feline viral leukaemia	Active Immunogen (HVF-1, CVF, PVF, *C. felis) and* Recombinant in Vector Virus (FeLV)	PureVax Feline 4 FeLV® FeLV	HVF-1 strain F-2 ≥ 10 $DICC^{4,9\ 50}$ CVF strains 431 and GI ≥ 2U ELISA PVF ≥ 10 $DICC^{3,550}$ *Chlamydia felis* strain 905 ≥ 10 $DIE^{3,0\ 50}$ FeLV recombinant canarypox vector Vcp ≥ 10 $DICC^{7,2\ 50}$
Feline viral leukaemia	Subunit recombinant	Leucogen	FeLV p45 at least 102µg (p45 fraction of gp 70)
	Inactivated virus	Leukocell 2	Multiple viral antigen vaccine (subgroups A, B, C and FOCMA antigen), produced from FeLV-transformed lymphoid cell line that releases soluble viral particles in cell culture medium.
	Virus Inactivated	Feline 2-FeLV ®	Contains tissue cultures, derived from FeLV, subgroups A and B. Viral antigens have been chemically inactivated.

6.7.6.3. SUGGESTIONS FOR A VACCINATION PROTOCOL

The American Animal Hospital Association (AAHA) published in 2020 a guide for the vaccination of cats (**Table 8**), which divides vaccines into core (recommended for all cats) and non-core (recommended based on an individualised risk/benefit assessment), so that vaccination protocols can be developed based on the risk factors of each patient, remembering to know the retroviral status prior to vaccination, since in positive cats it does not cause harm or the development of the disease, but neither does it generate any benefit, since vaccinating a positive cat or a cat whose retroviral status is unknown, may generate false expectations in the owners that may lead to questioning the efficiency of the vaccine if the disease finally occurs. (Aguilar B et al., 2019; Stone et al., 2020)..

Table 7. Vaccination guidelines for FeLV. Modified from (Aguilar B et al., 2019; Stone et al., 2020)..

<table>
<tr><td rowspan="2">Indoor cats</td><td rowspan="4">Inactivated or Recombinant FeLV Vaccine</td><td>Kittens (<16 weeks)</td><td>Cats >16 weeks (Unvaccinated)</td><td>Comments</td></tr>
<tr><td>Administer first dose at 8-9 weeks of age and booster 3-4 weeks later.

Finally 1 dose per year.</td><td>Administer 2 doses 3-4 weeks apart.

Subsequently 1 dose one year later.</td><td>It is recommended to know the retroviral status of the patient prior to vaccination.

Considered an essential vaccine for kittens and young adult cats under 1 year of age due to age-related susceptibility.

Considered a non-core vaccine for low-risk adult cats (no potential exposure to other FeLV+ cats or cats of unknown FeLV status).</td></tr>
<tr><td rowspan="2">Shelter cats</td><td>Less than 20 weeks old</td><td>Over 20 weeks old</td><td rowspan="2">It is recommended to know the retroviral status of the patient prior to vaccination.

Shelter: Positive cats should be separated from negative cats. Vaccination is recommended for cats kept in groups where their retroviral status is unknown.

Breeding: They must be free of FeLV, in which case vaccination is not required.</td></tr>
<tr><td>Administer first dose at 8-9 weeks of age and booster 3-4 weeks later.</td><td>Administer 2 doses 3-4 weeks apart.</td></tr>
</table>

7. CONCLUSION

Based on the information gathered in this work, we can conclude that several factors influence the outcome of FeLV interaction with the host, but mainly the immune system will determine the outcome, since the control of viral infection involves the innate response and its magnitude and quality is involved in the subsequent adaptive response, which determines the memory response. This interaction will determine the course of infection, and to achieve correct staging of the infection, it is important to know the duration of viraemia if present, and to know at what time the p27 antigen can be detected in blood, as this will help us to correctly use the POC and PCR tests. Cats that develop FeLV-associated disease are those with a weak or absent immune response, the virus affects a number of different apparatus and systems, and it is common to see tumours developing in different organs. Although there is no specific treatment for FeLV, rFeINF-ω has been used and patients have shown clinical improvement. Some of the mechanisms by which FeLV evades the immune response in some cats and how others have a better response against the virus remain to be elucidated, as the information available is old and there are not many current studies that continue to delve into the subject, this work could serve to arouse the curiosity of other researchers to continue delving into the subject.

8. REFERENCES

Abdollahi-Pirbazari, M., Jamshidi, S., Nassiri, S. M., & Zamani-Ahmadmahmudi, M. (2019). Comparative measurement of FeLV load in hemolymphatic tissues of cats with hematologic cytopenias. *BMC Veterinary Research*, *15*(1), 460. https://doi.org/10.1186/s12917-019-2208-y. https://doi.org/10.1186/s12917-019-2208-y

Abujamra, A. L., Akinsheye, I., Faller, D. V., Ghosh, S. K., Spanjaard, R. A., & Zhao, X. (2006). Leukemia virus long terminal repear activates NFkF pathway by a TLR-3 dependent mechanism. *Virology*, *345*(2), 390-403.

Ackley, C. D., Cooper, M. D., Dean, G. A., Donahue, P. R., Hoover, E. A., Mullins, J. I., ... Quackenbush, S. L. (1990). Lymphocyte Subset Alterations and Viral Determinants of Immunodeficiency Disease Induction by the Feline Leukemia Virus FeLV-FAIDS. *Journal of Virology*, *64*(11), 5465-5474.

Adams, P. W., Hebebrand, L. C., Hoover, E. A., Mathes, L. E., Nichols, W. S., Olsen, R. G., & Schaller, J. P. (1979). Immunosuppressive Properties of a Virion Polypeptide, a 15,000-Dalton Protein, from Feline Leukemia Virus. *Cancer Reserach*, *39*(3), 950-955.

Aguilar B, J., Autran de M, H., Basurto A, F. J., Flores, J. I., García, F., Garza, F., ... Lozano, I. G. (2019). Vaccination guidelines for Feline Viral Leukaemia COLAVAC-Mexico. *Vanguardia Veterinaria*(95), 50-52.

Ahmad, S., & Levy, L. S. (2010). The frequency of occurrence and nature of recombinant feline leukemia viruses in the induction of multicentric lymphoma by infection of the domestic cat with FeLV-945. *Virology*, *403*, 103-110.

Akira, S., & Uematsu, S. (2007). Toll-like Receptors and Type I Interferons. *Biological Chemistry*, *282*(21), 15319-15323.

Alsharifi, M., Müllbacher, A., & Regner, M. (2008). Interferon type I responses in primary and secondary infections. *Immunology and Cell Biology*(86), 239-245.

Argyl, D., Bain, D., Dunham, S., Golder, M. C., Hanlon, L., Jarret, O., ... Onions, D. E. (2001). Feline Leukemia Virus DNA Vaccine Efficacy Is Enhanced by Coadministration with Interleukin-12 (IL-12) and IL-18 Expression Vectors. *Journal of Virology*, *75*, 8424-8433.

Aroch, I., Ofri, R., & Sutton, G. A. (2008). Ocular Manifestations of Systemic Diseases. In *Slatter's Fundamentals of Veterinary Ophthalmology* (pp. 374-418). Copyright © 2008 Elsevier Inc. All rights reserved. https://doi.org/10.1016/b978-072160561-6.50021-6

Avallone, G., Boracchi, P., Caniatti, M., Forlani, A., Mortellaro, C. M., Roccabianca, P., & Santagostino, S. F. (2015). Feline Upper Respiratory Tract Lymphoma: Site, Cyto-histology, Phenotype, FeLV Expression, and Prognosis. *Veterinary pathology, 52*(2), 250-259.

Ballesteros, N., Collado, V. M., Doménech, A., Escolar, E., Gomez-Lucia, E., Martin, S., ... Sanjosé, L. (2011). Use of recombinant interferon omega in feline retrovirosis:From theory to practice. *Veterinary Immunology and Immunopathology*(143), 301-306.

Barret, K. E., Brooks, H., Boitano, S., & Barman, S. (2016). Immunity, Intection, & Inflammation. In K. E. Barret, H. Brooks, S. Boitano, & S. Barman (Eds.), *Ganong's Review Medical Physiology* (pp. 63-78). McGraw-Hill Education.

Benveniste, R. E., Sherr, C. J., & Todaro, G. J. (1975). Evolution of Type C Viral Genes: Origin of Feline Leukemia Virus. *SCIENCE, 190*, 886-888.

Benveniste, R. E., & Todaro, G. J. (1982). Gene transfer between eukaryotes. *SCIENCE, 217*, 1202.

Beyaert, R., Staal, J., & Vercammen, E. (2008). Viral Infection and Activation of Innate Immunology by Toll-Like Receptor 3. *Clinical Microbiology Reviews, 21*(1), 13-25.

Bjerve, K. S., Espevik, T., Kildahl-Andersen, O., & Nissen-Meyer, J. (1987). Effect of free fatty acids on the cytolytic activity of tumour necrosis factor/monocyte-derived cytotoxic factor. *Acta Pathol Microbiol Immunol Scand C, 95*(1), 21-26. https://doi.org/10.1111/j.1699-0463.1987.tb00004.x

Brown, M. A., Cunningham, M. W., Johnson, W. E., O'Brien, S. J., Roca, A. L., & Troyer, J. L. (2008). Genetic Characterization of Feline Leukemia Virus from Florida Panthers. *Emerging Infectious Diseases, 14*, 252-259.

Browne, E. P. (2020). The Role of Toll-Like Receptors in Retroviral Infection. *Microorganisms, 8*(11). https://doi.org/10.3390/microorganisms8111787

Calle R, J. F., Fernandéz G, L., Morales Z, L. M., & Ruiz S, J. (2013). Feline leukemia virus: a current pathogen requiring attention in Colombia. *Veterinaria y Zootecnia, 7*(2), 117-138.

Cattori, V., Gomes-Keller, M. A., Hofmann-Lehmann, R., Julhs, C., Lutz, H., Meli, M. L., ... Witting, B. (2011). The innate antiviral immune system of the cat: Molecular tools for the measurement of its state of activation. *Veterinary Immunology and Immunopathology, 143*(1-4), 209-281.

Cattori, V., Hofmann-Lehmann, R., Lutz, H., Niedererer, E., Pepin, A., Riond, B., . . . Willi, B. (2007a). Cellular segregation of feline leukemia provirus and viral RNA in leukocyte subsets of long-term experimentally infected cats. *Virus Research*(127), 9-16.

Cattori, V., Hofmann-Lehmann, R., Lutz, H., Niedererer, E., Pepin, A. C., Riond, B., ... Willi, B. (2007b). Cellular segregation of feline leukemia provirus and viral RNA in leukocyte subsets of long-term experimentally infected cats. *Virus Research*(127), 9-16.

Chang, H.-y., Gong, M.-j., Li, S.-f., Shao, J.-j., Xie, Y.-l., Zhao, F.-r., & Zhang, Y.-g. (2018). Type I Interferons: Distinct Biological Activities and Current Applications for Viral Infection. *Cellular Physiology and Biochemistry*, *3*(51), 2377-2396.

Chiu, E. S., Hoover, E. A., & Vanderwoude, S. (2018). Restropective Examination of Feline Leukemia Subgroup Characterization: Viral Interference Assay Deep Sequencing. *Viruses*, *10*(1), 1-12.

Colitz, C. M. (2005). Feline uveitis: diagnosis and treatment. *Clin Tech Small Anim Pract*, *20*(2), 117-120. https://doi.org/10.1053/j.ctsap.2004.12.016

Collado A, V. M. (2017). *In vitro* effect of type I on feline retrovirus expression and evaluation of its therapeutic application in naturally infected cats (Doctoral thesis). In. Madrid: Complutense University of Madrid.

Collado, V. M., Doménech, A., Escolar, E., Gómez-Lucía, E., Miró, G., Somsoles, M., & Tejerizo, G. (2007). Effect of type I interferons on the expression of feline leukaemia virus. *Veterinary Microbiology*, *123*, 180-186.

Collado, V. M., Doménech, A., Gómez-Lucía, E., & Miró, G. (2009). Effect of Type-I Interferon on Retroviruses. *Viruses*, *1*(3), 545-573.

Copelan, E. A., Rinehart, J. J., Lewis, M., Mathes, L., Olsen, R., & Sagone, A. (1983). The mechanism of retrovirus suppression of human T cell proliferation in vitro. *J Immunol*, *131*(4), 2017-2020.

Cotter, S. M. (1992). Feline leukemia virus: pathophysiology, prevention, and treatment. *Cancer Invest*, *10*(2), 173-181. https://doi.org/10.3109/07357909209032778

Couto, C. G. (2000). Advances in the treatment of the cat with lymphoma in practice. *J Feline Med Surg*, *2*(2), 95-100. https://doi.org/10.1053/jfms.2000.0079

Crawford, E. M., Davie, F., Jarret, W. F., & Martin, W. B. (1964). A Virus-like Particle associated with Leukaemia (Lymphosarcoma). *NATURE*, *202*, 567-568.

Day, M. J. (2012). *Clinical immunology of the dog and cat* (Second ed.). Manson Publishing.

Day, M. J., & Schultz, R. D. (2014). *Veterinary immunology - principles and practice* (Second ed.). Taylor & Francis Group.

Delgado Rodríguez, M., & Llorca Díaz, J. (2004). Longitudinal studies: concept and particularities. *Revista Española de Salud Pública*, *78*(2), 141-148.

Denner, J., Hübner, J., Jarret, O., Kurth, R., & Langhammer, S. (2010). Immunization with the transmembrane protein of a retrovirus, feline leukemia virus: Absence of antigenemia following challenge. *Antiviral Research*(89), 119-123.

Dezzutti, C. S., Wright, K. A., Lewis, M. G., Lafrado, L. J., & Olsen, R. G. (1989). FeLV-induced immunosuppression through alterations in signal transduction: Down regulation of protein kinase C. *Veterinary Immunology and Immunopathology*, *21*(1), 55-67. https://doi.org/https://doi.org/10.1016/0165-2427(89)90130-X

Essex, M., Grant, C. K., Cotter, S. M., & Hardy, W. D. (1981, 1981///). Role of Viruses in the Etiology of Naturally Occurring Feline Leukemia. Modern Trends in Human Leukemia IV, Berlin, Heidelberg.

Favrot, C., Wilhelm, S., Grest, P., Meli, M. L., Hofmann-Lehmann, R., & Kipar, A. (2005). Two cases of FeLV-associated dermatoses. *Vet Dermatol*, *16*(6), 407-412. https://doi.org/10.1111/j.1365-3164.2005.00480.x

Feschotte, C., & Gilbert, C. (2012). Endogenous viruses: insights into viral evolution and impact on host biology. *Nature Reviews Genetics*, *13*, 283-296.

Flynn, J. N., Dunham, S. P., Watson, V., & Jarrett, O. (2002). Longitudinal analysis of feline leukemia virus-specific cytotoxic T lymphocytes: correlation with recovery from infection. *J Virol*, *76*(5), 2306-2315. https://doi.org/10.1128/jvi.76.5.2306-2315.2002

Flynn, J. N., Hanlon, L., & Jarrett, O. (2000). Feline leukaemia virus: protective immunity is mediated by virus-specific cytotoxic T lymphocytes. *Immunology*, *101*(1), 120-125. https://doi.org/10.1046/j.1365-2567.2000.00089.x

Folks, T. M., Clouse, K. A., Justement, J., Rabson, A., Duh, E., Kehrl, J. H., & Fauci, A. S. (1989). Tumor necrosis factor alpha induces expression of human immunodeficiency virus in a chronically infected T-cell clone. *Proceedings of the National Academy of Sciences of the United States of America*, *86*(7), 2365-2368. https://doi.org/10.1073/pnas.86.7.2365

Ford, R. B., Gaskell, R. M., Hartmann, K., Hurley, K. F., Lappin, M. R., Levy, J. K., . . . Sparkes, A. H. (2013). 2013 AAFP Feline Vaccination Advisory Panel Report. (15), 785-808.

Frymus, T. (2017). *Maternally derived immunity and vaccination*. Retrieved 30/11/2020 from http://www.abcdcatsvets.org/maternally-derived-immunity-and-vaccination/

Fujino, Y., Ohno, K., & Tsujimoto, H. (2008). Molecular pathogenesis of feline leukemia virus-induced malignancies: Insertional mutagenesis. *Veterinary Immunology and Immunopathology*(123), 138-143.

Gasper, P. W., Hoover, E. A., Mullins, J. I., & Quackenbush, S. L. (1987). Experimental Transmission and Pathogenesis of Immunodeficiency Syndrome in Cats. *Blood*, *70*(6), 1880-1892.

Gelain, M. E., Antoniazzi, E., Bertazzolo, W., Zaccolo, M., & Comazzi, S. (2006). Chronic eosinophilic leukemia in a cat: cytochemical and immunophenotypical features.

Vet Clin Pathol, *35*(4), 454-459. https://doi.org/10.1111/j.1939-165x.2006.tb00164.x

Ginel Pérez, D. I., Maldonado Rivas, R., & Camacho Quesada, M. S. (1996). Immunosuppression diseases associated with feline leukaemia virus. *Clinica veterinaria de pequeños animales*, *16*(3), 142-164.

Glick, A. D., Horn, R. G., & Holscher, M. (1978). Characterization of feline glomerulonephritis associated with viral-induced hematopoietic neoplasms. *Am J Pathol*, *92*(2), 321-332.

Goh, C. R. (1990). Tumour necrosis factors in clinical practice. *Annals of the Academy of Medicine, Singapore*, *19*(2), 235-239.

Grant, C., Kipar, A., Kremendahl, J., Reinacher, M., & von Bothmer, I. (2000). Expression of Viral Proteins in Feline Leukemia Virus-associated Enteritis. *Veterinary Pathology*, *37*(2), 129-132.

Grosenbaugh, D. A., Frances-Duvert, V., Abedi, S., Feilmeier, B., Ru, H., & Poulet, H. (2017). Efficacy of a nonadjuvanted recombinant FeLV vaccine and two inactivated FeLV vaccines when subject to consistent virulent FeLV challenge conditions. *Biologicals*, *49*, 76-80. https://doi.org/10.1016/j.biologicals.2016.10.004

Gross, T. L., Clark, E. G., Hargis, A. M., Head, L. L., & Hainesh, D. M. (1993). Giant Cell Dermatosis in FeLV-positive Cats. *Veterinary Dermatology*, *4*(3), 117-122. https://doi.org/10.1111/j.1365-3164.1993.tb00204.x

Guliukina, I. A., Kucheruk, O. D., Komina, A. K., Zaberezhny, A. D., & Zhukovaand, E. V. (2019). Genetic diversity of feline leukemia virus. *OP Conf. Series: Earth and Environmental Science*, *315*, 1-4.

Guven, H., Konstantinidis, K. V., Alici, E., Aints, A., Abedi-Valugerdi, M., Christensson, B., ... Dilber, M. S. (2005). Efficient gene transfer into primary human natural killer cells by retroviral transduction. *Experimental Hematology*, *33*(11), 1320-1328. https://doi.org/https://doi.org/10.1016/j.exphem.2005.07.006

Harbour, D. A., Gunn-Moore, D. A., Gruffydd-Jones, T. J., Caney, S. M., Bradshaw, J., Jarrett, O., & Wiseman, A. (2002). Protection against oronasal challenge with virulent feline leukaemia virus lasts for at least 12 months following a primary course of immunisation with Leukocell 2 vaccine. *Vaccine*, *20*(23-24), 2866-2872. https://doi.org/10.1016/s0264-410x(02)00237-2

Hardy, W. (1993). Feline Oncoretroviruses. In *The retroviridae* (Vol. 2, pp. 109-180).

Hardy, W. D. (1981). Hematopoietic tumors of cats. *Journal of the American Animal Hospital Association*, *17*(6), 921-940.

Hardy, W. D. (1982). Immunopathology Induced by the Feline Leukemia Virus. *Springer Seminars in Immunopathology*, *5*(1), 75-106.

Hardy, W. D., Hess, P. W., MacEwen, E. G., McClelland, A. J., Zuckerman, E. E., Essex, M., ... Jarrett, O. (1976). Biology of Feline Leukemia Virus in the Natural Environment. *Cancer Research*, *36*(2 Part 2), 582.

Harris, D. T., Cianciolo, G. J., Snyderman, R., Argov, S., & Koren, H. S. (1987). Inhibition of human natural killer cell activity by a synthetic peptide homologous to a conserved region in the retroviral protein, p15E. *The Journal of Immunology*, *138*(3), 889-894. https://doi.org/10.4049/jimmunol.138.3.889

Hartman, K., & Sykes, J. E. (2014). Feline Leukemia Virus Infection. In J. E. Sykes (Ed.), *Canine and Feline Infectious Diseases (*1st ed., pp. 224-238). Saunders.

Hartmann (2012a). Clinical aspects of feline retroviruses: a review. *Viruses*, *4*(11), 2684-2710. https://doi.org/10.3390/v4112684

Hartmann (2012b). Feline Leukemia Virus Infection. In C. E. Greene & J. E. Sykes (Eds.), *Infectious Diseases of the Dog and Cat* (4th ed., pp. 108-135). Saunders.

Hartmann, K. (1998). Feline immunodeficiency virus infection: an overview. *Veterinary journal (London, England : 1997)*, *155*(2), 123-137. https://doi.org/10.1016/s1090-0233(98)80008-7

Hartmann, K. (2014). Feline Leukemia Virus Infection. In J. E. Sykes (Ed.), *Canine and Feline Infectious Diseases (*4th ed., pp. 108-136). Saunders.

Hartmann, K., & Hofmann-Lehmann, R. (2020). What's New in Feline Leukemia Virus Infection. *Veterinary Clinics: Small Animal Practice*, *50*(5), 1013-1036. https://doi.org/10.1016/j.cvsm.2020.05.006

Hause, W. R., Hoover, E. A., Olsen, R. G., Rojko, J. L., & Schaller, J. P. (1979). Detection of Feline Paraffin Embedding Leukemia Virus in Immunofluorescence Tissues of Cats Procedure. *Journal of the National Cancer Institute*(61), 1315-1321.

Heredia, J. M. (2019). Pathophysiopathogenesis of feline viral leukaemia. *Vanguardia veterinaria*(95), 8-10.

Hernández, J. C., Montoya, C. J., & Urcuqui-Inchima, S. (2007). Role of toll-like receptors in viral infections: HIV-1 as a model. *Biomedico*, *27*(2), 280-293.

Higgins, J., Hübscher, U., Lutz, H., Pedersen, N., Theilen, G., & Troy, F. A. (1980). Humoral Immune Reactivity to Feline Leukemia Virus and Associated Antigens in Cats Naturally Infected with Feline Leukemia Virus. *Cancer Reseach*, *40*, 3642-3651.

Higgins, R. J., Hinrinchs, S. H., D, S. M., Smith, M. O., & Torten, M. (1990). Type C retroviral expression in spontaneous feline olfactory neuroblastomas. *Acta Neuropathologica*, *80*(5), 547-583.

Hofmann-Lehmann, R., & Hartmann, K. (2020). Feline leukaemia virus infection: A practical approach to diagnosis. *J Feline Med Surg*, *22*(9), 831-846. https://doi.org/10.1177/1098612x20941785

Hoover, E. A., Mathiason, C. K., & Torres, A. N. (2005). Re-examination of feline leukemia virus: host relationships using real-time PCR. *Virology*, *332*(1), 272-283.

Hoover, E. A., Rojko, J. L., Wilson, P. L., & Olsen, R. G. (1981). Determinants of susceptibility and resistance to feline leukemia virus infection. I. Role of macrophages. *J Natl Cancer Inst*, *67*(4), 889-898. https://doi.org/10.1093/jnci/67.4.889

Horzinek, M. C. (1988). Feline Acquired Immunodeficiency Syndromes. In A. C. Beynen & H. A. Solleveld (Eds.), *New Developments in Biosciences: Their Implications for Laboratory Animal Science: Proceedings of the Third Symposium of the Federation of European Laboratory Animal Science Associations, held in Amsterdam, The Netherlands, 1-5 June 1987* (pp. 11-15). Springer Netherlands. https://doi.org/10.1007/978-94-009-3281-4_3

Jackson, M., Kipar, A., Kremendahl, J., & Reinacher, M. (2001). Comparative Examination of Cats with Feline Leukemia Virus-associated Enteritis and Other Relevant Forms of Feline Enteritis. *Veterinary pathology*, *38*(4), 359-371.

Jarret, O., & Russell, P. H. (1978). The occurrence of feline leukaemia virus neutralizing antibodies in cats. *International Journal of Cancer*(22), 351-357.

Jarrett, O., & Ganière, J. P. (1996). Comparative studies of the efficacy of a recombinant feline leukaemia virus vaccine. *Vet Rec*, *138*(1), 7-11. https://doi.org/10.1136/vr.138.1.7

Jarrett, W., Jarrett, O., Mackey, L., Laird, H., Hardy, W., Jr., & Essex, M. (1973). Horizontal Transmission of Leukemia Virus and Leukemia in the Cat. *JNCI: Journal of the National Cancer Institute*, *51*(3), 833-841. https://doi.org/10.1093/jnci/51.3.833

Kashiwa, H., Wright, S. C., & Bonavida, B. (1987). Regulation of B cell maturation and differentiation. I. Suppression of pokeweed mitogen-induced B cell differentiation by tumor necrosis factor (TNF). *J Immunol*, *138*(5), 1383-1390.

Khan, K. N. M. (1992). Role of the bone marrow microenvironment in the pathogenesis of feline leukemia virus-induced erythroid aplasia.

Khan, K. N. M., Kociba, G. J., & Wellman, M. L. (1993). Macrophage Tropism of Feline Leukemia Virus (FeLV) of Subgroup-C and Increased Production of Tumor Necrosis Factor-α by FeLV-Infected Macrophages. *Blood*, *81*(10), 2585-2590. https://doi.org/https://doi.org/10.1182/blood.V81.10.2585.2585

Kobilinsky, L., Hardy, W. D., Jr., Ellis, R., Witkin, S. S., & Day, N. K. (1980). In vitro activation of feline complement by feline leukemia virus. *Infect Immun*, *29*(1), 165-170. https://doi.org/10.1128/iai.29.1.165-170.1980

Kooistra, L. H., & Splitter, G. A. (1985). Killer cells of feline leukemia virus- and feline sarcoma virus-infected transformed cells: The role of NK, ADCC, and in vitro generated cytotoxic cells. *Cellular Immunology*, *94*(2), 466-479. https://doi.org/https://doi.org/10.1016/0008-8749(85)90271-0.

Krause, C. D., Pestka, S., & Walter, M. R. (2004). Interferons, interferon-like cytokines and their receptors. *Immunological Reviews*, *202*, 8-32.

Lafrado, L. J., & Olsen, R. G. (1986). Demonstration of depressed polymorphonuclear leukocyte function in nonviremic FeLV-infected cats. *Cancer Invest*, *4*(4), 297-300. https://doi.org/10.3109/07357908609017509

Langhammer, S., Fiebig, U., Kurth, R., & Denner, J. (2005). Neutralising antibodies against the transmembrane protein of feline leukaemia virus (FeLV). *Vaccine*, *23*(25), 3341-3348. https://doi.org/10.1016/j.vaccine.2005.01.091

Langhammer, S., Fiebig, U., Kurth, R., & Denner, J. (2011). Increased neutralizing antibody response after simultaneous immunization with leukogen and the feline leukemia virus transmembrane protein. *Intervirology*, *54*(2), 78-86. https://doi.org/10.1159/000318892

Langhammer, S., Hübner, J., Kurth, R., & Denner, J. (2006). Antibodies neutralizing feline leukaemia virus (FeLV) in cats immunized with the transmembrane envelope protein p15E. *Immunology*, *117*(2), 229-237. https://doi.org/10.1111/j.1365-2567.2005.02291.x

Leal, R. O., & Gil, S. (2016). The Use of Recombinant Feline Interferon Omega Therapy as an Immune-Modulator in Cats Naturally Infected with Feline Immunodeficiency Virus: New Perspectives. *Veterinary Sciences*, *3*(4).

Lehmann, R., Joller, H., Haagmans, B. L., & Lutz, H. (1992). Tumor necrosis factor alpha levels in cats experimentally infected with feline immunodeficiency virus: effects of immunization and feline leukemia virus infection. *Vet Immunol Immunopathol*, *35*(1-2), 61-69. https://doi.org/10.1016/0165-2427(92)90121-6

Levy, L. S. (2008). Advances in understanding molecular determinants in FeLV pathology. *Veterinary immunology and immunopathology*(123), 14-22.

Lewis, M. G., Kociba, G. J., Rojko, J. L., Stiff, M. I., Haberman, A. B., Velicer, L. F., & Olsen, R. G. (1985). Retroviral-associated eosinophilic leukemia in the cat. *Am J Vet Res*, *46*(5), 1066-1070.

Linenberger, M. L., & Deng, T. (1999). The effects of feline retroviruses on cytokine expression. *Veterinary Immunology and Immunopathology*, *72*(3), 343-368. https://doi.org/https://doi.org/10.1016/S0165-2427(99)00147-6

Little, S., Levy, J., Hartmann, K., Hofmann-Lehmann, R., Hosie, M., Olah, G., & Denis, K. S. (2020). 2020 AAFP Feline Retrovirus Testing and Management Guidelines. *J Feline Med Surg*, *22*(1), 5-30. https://doi.org/10.1177/1098612x19895940

Littwitz-Salomon, E., Dittmer, U., & Sutter, K. (2016). Insufficient natural killer cell responses against retroviruses: how to improve NK cell killing of retrovirus-infected cells. *Retrovirology*, *13*(1), 77. https://doi.org/10.1186/s12977-016-0311-8

Littwitz-Salomon, E., Malyshkina, A., Schimmer, S., & Dittmer, U. (2018). The Cytotoxic Activity of Natural Killer Cells Is Suppressed by IL-10(+) Regulatory T Cells During Acute Retroviral Infection. *Front Immunol*, *9*, 1947. https://doi.org/10.3389/fimmu.2018.01947. https://doi.org/10.3389/fimmu.2018.01947

Luaces, I., Doménech, A., García-Montijano, M., Collado, V. M., Sánchez, C., German, T., ... Gómez-Lucía, E. (2008). Detection of Feline Leukemia Virus in the Endangered Iberian Lynx (*Lynx Pardinus*). *J Vet Diagn Invest*, *20*, 381-385.

Lähdevirta, J., Maury, C. P., Teppo, A. M., & Repo, H. (1988). Elevated levels of circulating cachectin/tumor necrosis factor in patients with acquired immunodeficiency syndrome. *Am J Med*, *85*(3), 289-291. https://doi.org/10.1016/0002-9343(88)90576-1

López-Goñi, I. (2015). We are what we are because we are viruses and bacteria: the impact of endogenous microorganisms on host biology. *NACC. Bioloxia*, *22*, 15-21.

Mach, B., Steimle, V., Martinez-Soria, E., & Reith, W. (1996). REGULATION OF MHC CLASS II GENES: Lessons from a Disease. *Annual Review of Immunology*, *14*(1), 301-331. https://doi.org/10.1146/annurev.immunol.14.1.301

Malinowski, C. (2006). Canine and Feline Nasal Neoplasia. *Clinical Techniques in Small Animal Practice*, *21*(2), 89-94. https://doi.org/https://doi.org/10.1053/j.ctsap.2005.12.016

Mathes, L. E., Olsen, R. G., Hebebrand, L. C., Hoover, E. A., Schaller, J. P., Adams, P. W., & Nichols, W. S. (1979). Immunosuppressive Properties of a Virion Polypeptide, a 15,000-Dalton Protein, from Feline Leukemia Virus. *Cancer Research*, *39*(3), 950.

Maury, C. P., & Lăhdevirta, J. (1990). Correlation of serum cytokine levels with haematological abnormalities in human immunodeficiency virus infection. *J Intern Med*, *227*(4), 253-257. https://doi.org/10.1111/j.1365-2796.1990.tb00154.x

Mims, C. A. (1964). ASPECTS OF THE PATHOGENESIS OF VIRUS DISEASES. *Bacteriological reviews*, *28*(1), 30-71.

Mizayawa, T. (2002). Feline leukemia virus and Feline Immunodeficiency virus. *Frontiers in Bioscience: a journal and virtual library*, *4*(7), 504-518.

Modiano, J. F. (2013). The Etiology of Cancer. In *Withrow & MacEwen's Small Animal Clinical oncology* (5th ed., pp. 1-26). Saunders.

Mogensen, S. C. (1979). Role of macrophages in natural resistance to virus infections. *Microbiological reviews*, *43*(1), 1-26.

Montaraz C, J. A. (2012). Innate Immunity. In *Introduction to Immunology (*2nd ed., pp. 19-30). UNAM Cuautitlán.

MSD (2023). *NOBIVAC® FELINE 2-FeLV*. Retrieved 9 March from https://www.msd-salud-animal.mx/productos/nobivac-feline-2-felv-2/

Murphy, B. (2016). Retroviridae. In E. J. Dubovi & J. N. MacLachlan (Eds.), *Fenner's Veterinary Virology (*pp. 270-297). Academic Press.

Nagata, M., & Rosenkrantz, W. (2013). Cutaneous viral dermatoses in dogs and cats. *Compend Contin Educ Vet*, *35*(7), E1.

Neil, J. C. (2010). Feline Leukemia and Sarcoma Viruses. In B. W. Mahy & M. H. Regenmortel (Eds.), *Desk encyclopedia of animal and bacterial virology* (pp. 283-287). Elsevier.

News, B. (2019). Feline leukaemia. *Veterinary Vanguard*, *95*, 42-44.

O'Neil, L. L., Burkhard, M. J., & Hoover, E. A. (1996). Frequent perinatal transmission of feline immunodeficiency virus by chronically infected cats. *Journal of virology*, *70*(5), 2894-2901. https://doi.org/10.1128/JVI.70.5.2894-2901.1996

Odeh, M. (1990). The role of tumour necrosis factor-alpha in acquired immunodeficiency syndrome. *J Intern Med*, *228*(6), 549-556. https://doi.org/10.1111/j.1365-2796.1990.tb00278.x

Ogilvie, G. K., Tompkins, M. B., & Tompkins, W. A. F. (1988). Clinical and immunologic aspects of FeLV-induced immunosuppression. *Veterinary Microbiology*, *17*(3), 287-296. https://doi.org/https://doi.org/10.1016/0378-1135(88)90070-3

Orosz, C. G., Zinn, N. E., Olsen, R. G., & Mathes, L. E. (1985). Retrovirus-mediated immunosuppression. II. FeLV-UV alters in vitro murine T lymphocyte behavior by reversibly impairing lymphokine secretion. *J Immunol*, *135*(1), 583-590.

Pacitti, A. M., Jarrett, O., & Hay, D. (1986). Transmission of feline leukaemia virus in the milk of a non-viraemic cat. *Vet Rec*, *118*(14), 381-384. https://doi.org/10.1136/vr.118.14.381

Palmero, M. L., & Carballés Pérez, V. (2010). Feline leukaemia. In *Feline infectious diseases (*pp. 5-90). SERVET.

Paoletti, E. (1996). Applications of pox virus vectors to vaccination: an update. *Proceedings of the National Academy of Sciences*, *93*(21), 11349-11353. https://doi.org/10.1073/pnas.93.21.11349

Patel, M., Carritt, K., Lane, J., Jayappa, H., Stahl, M., & Bourgeois, M. (2015). Comparative Efficacy of Feline Leukemia Virus (FeLV) Inactivated Whole-Virus Vaccine and Canarypox Virus-Vectored Vaccine during Virulent FeLV Challenge and Immunosuppression. *Clinical and Vaccine Immunology*, *22*(7), 798-805. https://doi.org/10.1128/CVI.00034-15

Pedersen, N. C. (1993). Immunogenicity and efficacy of a commercial feline leukemia virus vaccine. *J Vet Intern Med*, *7*(1), 34-39. https://doi.org/10.1111/j.1939-1676.1993.tb03166.x

Porras M, R. (2007). Role of cytokines in feline leukaemia virus infection. In (Vol. 1, pp. 584-596). Madrid: Revistas Complutense de Ciencias Veterinarias.

Poulet, H., Brunet, S., Boularand, C., Guiot, A. L., Leroy, V., Tartaglia, J., ... Desmettre, P. (2003). Efficacy of a canarypox virus-vectored canarypox vaccine against feline leukaemia [https://doi.org/10.1136/vr.153.5.141]. *Veterinary Record*, *153*(5), 141-145. https://doi.org/https://doi.org/10.1136/vr.153.5.141

Puig-Basagoti, F., & Saíz, J. C. (2001). Subgenomic replicons of hepatitis C virus (HCV): new expectations for hepatitis C prophylaxis and treatment. *Gastroenterology and Hepatology*, *24*(10), 506-510.

Quiroz, J. (2019). Ocular alterations related to feline viral leukaemia virus. *Vanguardia veterinaria*(95), 32-34.

Ramírez, H., Autran, M., García, M. M., Carmona, M., Rodríguez, C., & Martínez, H. A. (2016). Genotyping of feline leukemia virus in Mexican housecats. *Arch Virol*, *161*(4), 1039-1045. https://doi.org/10.1007/s00705-015-2740-4

Rees, C. A., & Goldschmidt, M. H. (1998). Cutaneous horn and squamous cell carcinoma in situ (Bowen's disease) in a cat. *J Am Anim Hosp Assoc*, *34*(6), 485-486. https://doi.org/10.5326/15473317-34-6-485

Reinacher, M. (1989). Diseases Associated with Spontaneous Feline Leukemia Virus (FeLV) Infection in Cats. *Veterinary Immunology and Immunopathology*(21), 85-95.

Rideout, B. A., Moore, P. F., & Pedersen, N. C. (1992). Persistent upregulation of MHC Class II antigen expression on T-lymphocytes from cats experimentally infected with feline immunodeficiency virus. *Veterinary Immunology and Immunopathology*, *35*(1), 71-81. https://doi.org/https://doi.org/10.1016/0165-2427(92)90122-7

Rojko, J. L., Hoover, E. A., Mathes, L. E., Olsen, R. G., & Schaller, J. P. (1979). Pathogenesis of experimental feline leukemia virus infection. *J Natl Cancer Inst*, *63*(3), 759-768. https://doi.org/10.1093/jnci/63.3.759

Rojko, J. L., Hoover, E. A., Quackenbush, S. L., & Olsen, R. G. (1982). Reactivation of latent feline leukaemia virus infection. *Nature*, *298*(5872), 385-388. https://doi.org/10.1038/298385a0

Rossi, F., Aresu, L., Martini, V., Trez, D., Zanetti, R., Coppola, L. M., ... Zini, E. (2019). Immune-complex glomerulonephritis in cats: a retrospective study based on clinico-pathological data, histopathology and ultrastructural features. *BMC Veterinary Research*, *15*(1), 303. https://doi.org/10.1186/s12917-019-2046-y. https://doi.org/10.1186/s12917-019-2046-y.

Schubach, T. M., Schubach, A., Okamoto, T., Barros, M. B., Figueiredo, F. B., Cuzzi, T., ... Wanke, B. (2004). Evaluation of an epidemic of sporotrichosis in cats: 347 cases (1998-2001). *J Am Vet Med Assoc*, *224*(10), 1623-1629. https://doi.org/10.2460/javma.2004.224.1623.

Schultz, R. D., Scott, F. W., Duncan, J. R., & Gillespie, J. H. (1974). Feline immunoglobulins. *Infection and immunity*, *9*(2), 391-393. https://doi.org/10.1128/IAI.9.2.391-393.1974

Scott, F. W., Csiza, C. K., & Gillespie, J. H. (1970). Maternally derived immunity to feline panleukopenia. *J Am Vet Med Assoc*, *156*(4), 439-453.

Sehn, J. K. (2015). Insertions and deletions (Indels). In S. Kulkarni & J. Pfeifer (Eds.), *Clinical Genomics* (1st ed., pp. 130-148). Academic Press.

Sellon, R. K., Jordan, H. L., Kennedy-Stoskopf, S., Tompkins, M. B., & Tompkins, W. A. (1994). Feline immunodeficiency virus can be experimentally transmitted via milk during acute maternal infection. *J Virol*, *68*(5), 3380-3385. https://doi.org/10.1128/jvi.68.5.3380-3385.1994

Sen, G. C. (2001). Viruses and Interferons. *Annual Review of Microbiology*, *55*, 255-281.

Sharifi, H., Nassiri, S. M., Esmaelli, H., & Khoshnegah, J. (2007). Eosinophilic leukaemia in a cat. *Journal of Feline Medicine & Surgery*, *9*(6), 514-517. https://doi.org/https://doi.org/10.1016/j.jfms.2007.05.004

Sherwin, S. A., Benveniste, R. E., & Todaro, G. J. (1978). Complement-mediated lysis of type-C virus: effect of primate and human sera on various retroviruses. *Int J Cancer*, *21*(1), 6-11. https://doi.org/10.1002/ijc.2910210103

Souza, H., Da Costa, F., Dorigon, O., Damico, C., & Brito, M. (2010). Multiple cutaneous horns on the footpads of a persian cat. *Ciência Rural*, *40*, 678-681.

St Denis, K. A. (2022). Feline Leukemia Virus Disease. *MSD Manual Veterinary manual*.

Stone, A. E., Brummet, G. O., Carozza, E. M., Kass, P. H., Petersen, E. P., Sykes, J., & Westman, M. E. (2020). 2020 AAHA/AAFP Feline Vaccination Guidelines. *J Feline Med Surg*, *22*(9), 813-830. https://doi.org/10.1177/1098612x20941784

Stützer, B., Müller, F., Majzoub, M., Lutz, H., Greene, C. E., Hermanns, W., & Hartmann, K. (2010). Role of latent feline leukemia virus infection in nonregenerative cytopenias of cats. *J Vet Intern Med*, *24*(1), 192-197. https://doi.org/10.1111/j.1939-1676.2009.0417.x

Sánchez Pacheco, A. (2019). Feline viral leukaemia vaccination. *Vanguardia veterinaria*(95), 46-48.

Tuomari, D. L., Olsen, R. G., Singh, V. K., & Kraut, E. H. (1984). Detection of circulating immune complexes by a Clq/protein A-ELISA during the preneoplastic stages of feline leukemia virus infection. *Veterinary Immunology and Immunopathology*, *7*(3), 227-238. https://doi.org/https://doi.org/10.1016/0165-2427(84)90081-3

Vega Robledo, G. B. (2009). Major histocompatibility complex. *Revista de la Facultad de Medicina UNAM*, *52*(2), 86-88.

Vieira, V. A., Herbert, N., Cromhout, G., Adland, E., & Goulder, P. (2022). Role of Early Life Cytotoxic T Lymphocyte and Natural Killer Cell Immunity in Paediatric HIV Cure/Remission in the Anti-Retroviral Therapy Era [Review]. *Frontiers in Immunology*, *13*.

Wardini, A. B., Guimarães-Costa, A. B., Nascimento, M. T., Nadaes, N. R., Danelli, M. G., Mazur, C., ... Pinto-da-Silva, L. H. (2010). Characterization of neutrophil extracellular traps in cats naturally infected with feline leukemia virus. *J Gen Virol*, *91*(Pt 1), 259-264. https://doi.org/10.1099/vir.0.014613-0

Welsh, R. M., Jr., Jensen, F. C., Cooper, N. R., & Oldstone, M. B. (1976). Inactivation of lysis of oncornaviruses by human serum. *Virology*, *74*(2), 432-440. https://doi.org/10.1016/0042-6822(76)90349-4

Willet, B. J., & Hoise, M. J. (2013). Feline Leukaemia Virus: Half a century since its discovery. *The Veterinary Journal*, *195*, 16-23.

Wonderling, R., Powell, T., Baldwin, S., Morales, T., Snyder, S., Keiser, K., ... Milhausen, M. (2002). Cloning, expression, purification, and biological activity of five feline type I interferons. *Veterinary Immunology and Immunopathology*, *89*(1), 13-27. https://doi.org/https://doi.org/10.1016/S0165-2427(02)00188-5.

Wooley, D. P., Peterson, K. T., Taylor, R. J., Paul, C. C., & Baumann, M. A. (2000). Strain-dependent productive infection of a unique eosinophilic cell line by human immunodeficiency virus type 1. *AIDS Res Hum Retroviruses*, *16*(14), 1405-1415. https://doi.org/10.1089/08892220050140955

Yasmin, A. P., Melissa, J. B., Julie, K. L., Michael, M., Natascha, T. H., Brian, J. W., & Margaret, J. H. (2021). Measuring the Humoral Immune Response in Cats Exposed to Feline Leukaemia Virus [article]. *Viruses*, *13*(428), 428-428. https://doi.org/10.3390/v13030428

Yuhki, N., Mullikin, J. C., Beck, T., Stephens, R., & O'Brien, S. J. (2008). Sequences, Annotation and Single Nucleotide Polymorphism of the Major Histocompatibility Complex in the Domestic Cat. *PLOS ONE*, *3*(7), e2674. https://doi.org/10.1371/journal.pone.0002674

Zachary, J. F. (2012). Mechanims of Microbial Infections. In D. McGavin & J. F. Zachary (Eds.), *Pathologic Basis of Veterinary Disease* (5th ed., pp. 147-240). Mosby, Inc.

Zachary, J. F. (2017). Mechanims of Microbial Infections. In J. F. Zachary (Ed.), *Pathologic Basis of Veterinary Disease* (6th ed., pp. 132-241). Elsevier.

Zoetis (2023). *Leukocell® 2 Feline Viral Leukaemia Vaccine*. Retrieved 5 March from https://www.zoetis.mx/products/gatos/leukocell-2.aspx

Zucali, J. R., Broxmeyer, H. E., Dinarello, C. A., Gross, M. A., & Weiner, R. S. (1987). Regulation of early human hematopoietic (BFU-E and CFU-GEMM) progenitor cells in vitro by interleukin 1-induced fibroblast-conditioned medium. *Blood*, *69*(1), 33-37.

ACKNOWLEDGEMENTS

The present review was supervised by the different experts in the area of Virology, genetics and Molecular Biology, as well as specialists in veterinary Systemic Pathology: Drs. Vianey Ramirez Andoney, Alejandro Vargas Ruiz, Ernesto Marin Flamand and Humberto Alejandro Martinez Rodriguez.

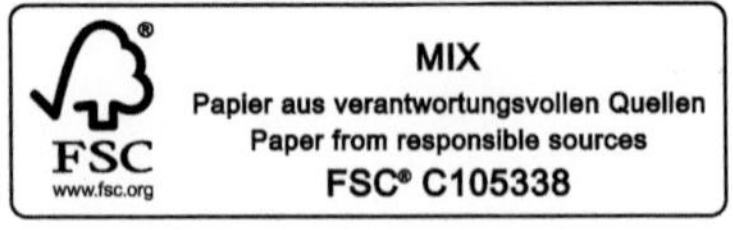

Printed by Books on Demand GmbH, Norderstedt / Germany